READING FOR HEALTH

Series in Victorian Studies

Joseph McLaughlin, series editor

Katherine D. Harris, *Forget Me Not: The Rise of the British Literary Annual, 1823–1835*

Rebecca Rainof, *The Victorian Novel of Adulthood: Plot and Purgatory in Fictions of Maturity*

Erika Wright, *Reading for Health: Medical Narratives and the Nineteenth-Century Novel*

Daniel Bivona and Marlene Tromp, editors, *Culture and Money in the Nineteenth Century: Abstracting Economics*

Reading for Health

Medical Narratives and the Nineteenth-Century Novel

Erika Wright

OHIO UNIVERSITY PRESS ATHENS, OHIO

Ohio University Press, Athens, Ohio 45701
ohioswallow.com

Printed in the United States of America
Ohio University Press books are printed on acid-free paper ∞ ™

26 25 24 23 22 21 20 19 18 17 16 5 4 3 2 1

Library of Congress Cataloging-in-Publication Data

Names: Wright, Erika, 1970– author.
Title: Reading for health : medical narratives and the nineteenth-century novel / Erika Wright.
Description: Athens, Ohio : Ohio University Press, [2016] | Series: Series in Victorian studies | Includes bibliographical references and index.
Identifiers: LCCN 2015041247| ISBN 9780821422243 (hc : alk. paper) | ISBN 9780821445631 (pdf)
Subjects: LCSH: English fiction—19th century—History and criticism. | Literature and medicine—Great Britain—History—19th century. | Medicine in literature.
Classification: LCC PR878.M42 W75 2016 | DDC 823/.8093561–dc23
LC record available at http://lccn.loc.gov/2015041247

For Ted and Devin

Contents

Acknowledgments

Like staying healthy, writing a book takes sustained effort and tremendous discipline. And when that fails, it takes a little luck and a lot of outside support. I am grateful for the opportunity to thank the many people whose advice, encouragement, and humor appear in the pages of this book. My first debt of gratitude goes to Hilary Schor, who devoted countless hours and attention to my work, challenging me to read and think more deeply and inspiring me to write with passion and conviction. Her words and influence are present throughout this book. I want to thank Jim Kincaid for guiding me with his wit and unconventional wisdom, both of which broadened my understanding of Victorian culture and altered my conception of our own. For her insight and encouragement, I offer my sincerest gratitude to Emily Anderson. Our numerous conversations allowed me to see more clearly my vision for this project. Meg Russett read (and reread) the manuscript, offering guidance that helped me clarify my aims and assert my authority. I am grateful to Jonathan Grossman, who, at a crucial moment, transformed my thinking about the book, allowing me to understand the larger stakes of the story I was trying to tell. My heartfelt thanks must go to Joe Boone. His brilliance, friendship, and, above all, unwavering confidence in this project sustained me throughout this process.

I am fortunate to have a strong and extended network of friends, family, and colleagues who have supported me (personally and professionally) along the way. John Jordan, Philippa Levine, Theresa Mangum, Tania Modleski, Susan Zeiger, and the whole cast of The Dickens Universe provided valuable advice early on when I was still figuring out what to make of illness and health in the Victorian novel. For their thoughtful comments on dissertation chapters, conference papers, book proposals, and manuscript drafts, and for making me laugh, I want to thank Michael Blackie, Leslie Bruce, David Namie, Pamela Schaff, Jeff Solomon, Kathryn Strong Hansen, Alice Villaseñor, and Annalisa Zox-Weaver. I am especially grateful to Beth Callaghan for always being a thoughtful reader and listener, and to Becky Woomer for knowing just what to say and how best to say it. Their scholarly advice and parenting wisdom have served me well. To my mother, Kristin Wright, I owe perhaps the most for always seeing the best in what I do.

The funding I received from the University of Southern California's English Department and Gender Studies Department, the Marta Feuchtwanger Foundation, the Philadelphia College of Physicians, and the Huntington Library provided me with the time and resources to research and complete this project. It has been a great pleasure to work with Joseph McLaughlin, Rick Huard, Nancy Basmajian, and Sally Bennett Boyington at Ohio University Press. I am also indebted to Pamela Gilbert for her support of this book and for her scholarship, which has greatly influenced my thinking about Victorian health. I truly appreciate the careful consideration of the anonymous reader of the manuscript and the reader for *Studies in the Novel*, where a portion of chapter 1 first appeared as pages 377–94 in volume 42, no. 4 (2010) and is reprinted with permission by Johns Hopkins University Press.

Finally, the book would not be half as meaningful to me without the love and companionship of Ted Johnson, who has been part of this project from the beginning, and Devin Johnson, who came along at just the right time. I dedicate this book to them. They have enriched my own story beyond measure.

Introduction

Becoming Patient Readers

> In modern stories prepared for more refined or fastidious audiences than those of [Charles] Dickens, the funereal excitement is obtained, for the most part, not by the infliction of violent or—disgusting death; but in the suspense, the pathos, and the more or less by all felt, and recognized, phenomena of the sick-room. The temptation, to weak writers, of this order of subject is especially great, because the study of it from the living—or dying—model is so easy, and to many has been the most impressive part of their own personal experience.
>
> —John Ruskin, "Fiction, Fair and Foul" (1880)

> The pleasures of health are taken as a matter of course, and are only passively appreciated.
>
> —Alexander Shand, "The Pleasures of Sickness" (1889)

Readers of Victorian novels will likely appreciate John Ruskin's critique of "modern stories." Disease and death are everywhere in nineteenth-century novels. Imagine Charles Dickens's *Bleak House* (1853) without Esther Summerson's delirium or the fetid atmosphere of Tom-All-Alone's, Charlotte Brontë's *Jane Eyre* (1847) without a young Jane clutching a dead Helen Burns, or an Elizabeth Gaskell novel without industrial illness—whether Mary Barton's inanition or the fluff in little Bessy's lungs. For many scholars, the Victorian novel would not be *Victorian* without illness.[1] As Miriam Bailin observes in *The Sickroom in Victorian Fiction: The Art of Being Ill*, "There is scarcely a Victorian fictional narrative without its ailing protagonist, its depiction of a sojourn in the sickroom."[2] But for Ruskin, these "sojourns" are morally and aesthetically suspect—the mark of a lazy writer. Not only do such scenes cater to the reader's baser instincts,[3] but they also, perhaps more damningly, take minimal effort and almost no talent to depict. "Few authors of second or third rate genius," Ruskin argues, "can either record or invent a probable conversation in ordinary life; but few, on the other hand, are so destitute of observant faculty as to be unable to chronicle the broken syllables and languid movements of an invalid" (*Works*, 274).

Disappointed by what he saw as an unfortunate dependence on the morbid and the pathological in the fiction of his day, Ruskin called for a return to a healthier literature, one in which the death toll is kept at a minimum, the sickroom scene is understated or absent, and the characters are not so morally repugnant. Ruskin identifies the various deaths in Dickens's *Bleak House* and the unredeemable characters in George Eliot's *Mill on the Floss* (1860) as particularly objectionable. By way of contrast, Sir Walter Scott's novels—which as Ruskin notes favor "character[s] of a highly virtuous and lofty stamp" (*Works*, 285), "landscape[s] [that are] rich" (378), intricately woven plots, and a laudable purpose, which is to "study the effects of true and false religion on conduct" (381)—exemplify the "healthy and helpful literature" (376) for which Ruskin was nostalgic. But even Scott was not completely immune to the allure of sickbeds. Ruskin cites *St. Ronan's Well* (1824), *The Fair Maid of Perth* (1828), and *Castle Dangerous* (1832), which were written during the period of illness before Scott's death,[4] as having sunk "into fellowship with the normal disease which festers throughout the whole body of our lower fictitious literature" (276). Disease, for Ruskin, was literal and metaphorical—the one often sliding into the other. Although a writer need not be unhealthy to write sick literature, those who suffer from actual illnesses are presumably more likely to succumb to the reading public's prurient desire for "vice and gloom" (276) and to feature an array of diseased characters and insalubrious situations. "No good is ever done to society," Ruskin explains, "by the pictorial representation of its diseases" (376).

Ruskin was not the only critic who thought about literature this way. As Bruce Haley points out in his seminal study *The Healthy Body and Victorian Culture,* "The Victorian critic believed that he should diagnose a work, looking for signs of disease or soundness, then looking further for causes of the disclosed condition."[5] For example, when Thomas Carlyle writes about Rousseau in 1841, he claims that Rousseau's "books[,] like himself, are what I call unhealthy; not the good sort of Book."[6] In his 1858 analysis of Scott's Waverley novels, Walter Bagehot implies—as Ruskin would much later—that the author's experience with literal health was somehow integral to literary form, particularly when it comes to depicting monstrous or "anomalous" characters. Bagehot lauds Scott's superior skills of characterization, claiming, "A writer must have sympathy with health before he can show us how and where and to what extent that which is unhealthy deviates from it."[7]

Literary criticism that aligns the author's mental, physical, and moral health with the metaphorical soundness of his text—though common enough during the nineteenth century—represents a type of evaluative and biographical analysis that has largely fallen out of favor. Twentieth- and twenty-first-century scholars are much less inclined to make claims about the role that an author's health plays in the value of his or her work.[8] But in turning away from such health claims, we have, I suggest, lost a chance to see the subtle ways in which health—particularly physical health—operates in these works: the challenges it poses and the reading practices it engenders.

Ruskin suggests in the above epigraph that illness is "impressive"—that one's experience with illness makes an impression on her life in a way that the experience of health cannot. Narratively speaking, health functions as little more than an addendum to the story of illness; it becomes simply a charming (or annoying) resolution, an innocuous character trait, or a pernicious metaphor for all that is right and good. In "Pathologizing the Victorians," Kirstie Blair comments on the scholarly interest in disease at the 2000 Victorian Institute Conference on Victorian illness, health, and medicine, observing, "Almost every speaker focuse[d] on illness rather than health" and "Pathology has been the focus of Victorian criticism for some time."[9] Medical historian Roger Cooter makes a similar point in a 2003 review for *Victorian Studies:* "Corporeality and pathology have become obligatory points of passage in the study of Victorian society and culture."[10] Over a decade later, this preoccupation is still largely the case,[11] for although we may be somewhat less interested than the Victorians in judging a novel based on how the writer felt as she wrote, we continue to ask why sickness is so pervasive and what exactly disease means in Victorian novels and to the Victorians themselves.[12]

My reading of the Victorian novel draws from these two critical modes: first, the current scholarly interest in disease, and second, the nineteenth-century call for "healthy literature." I am sympathetic to our persistent fascination in Victorian studies with the pathological, and I am inspired by the methods recent scholars have used to articulate the social, political, and narrative implications of illness. But I am equally intrigued by Ruskin's frustration with the ample material Victorian writers left us. I do not aim, as Ruskin did, to condemn the Victorian writers' gratuitous use of illness, nor do I want to use sickness as a barometer for evaluating their characters. I do, however, want to ask, "Why always disease?" In asking this question, I want to suggest that health is an epistemological problem and that nineteenth-century narratives register, through both their form and their content, the difficulty of knowing what health is, how to preserve it, and whose is best.[13] These questions are made explicit in the periodical press, in government pamphlets, and in memoirs, and are implicit as well as explicit in novels.[14]

One reason for the critical interest in disease, of course, is that disease and illness are medically and narratively more interesting than health. To use Ruskin's term, illness is "impressive," whereas health is, as Alexander Shand notes in the second epigraph to this introduction, a "matter of course," only "passively appreciated." Health is, in other words, a nonstory. Like Athena Vrettos, who points out in *Somatic Fictions* (1995) that "[t]o be ill is to produce narrative,"[15] John Wiltshire surmises in his work on Jane Austen, "If the healthy body is largely passive, unconscious of itself, then the unhealthy body, as a site of anxious self-concentration, is the source of events, of narrative energies."[16] For the doctor, illness is a problem *to solve;* it must be diagnosed, treated, and cured. For the patient, illness is an obstacle *to overcome* or perhaps a punishment for sin. Indeed, illness forces us to take notice of our bodies and behaviors, to experience compassion, to purge, to repent. In contrast, health signifies the absence of all of this; if anything, it functions merely as the end of the action, the prized reward. It provides the requisite closure or the inaugurating condition that incites narrative, but it is certainly not what keeps the story going.

Robert James's definition of health in his three-volume *A Medicinal Dictionary* (1743–45)[17] attests to the unconsciousness that attends health: the body is in a "sound state," he explains, when "nothing is wanting" (lxvi). James depicts health as a negation or an absence ("nothing is wanting") rather than an affirmation or presence (that is, "every need is met"). Borrowing from D. A. Miller, whose work has greatly influenced this book, we might describe health as the nonnarratable state of "quiescence assumed by a novel before the beginning and supposedly *recovered* by it at the end."[18] But even here, we can see just how pervasive the disease narrative is, for the very form of the traditional novel and the language we use to theorize it rely on a reading of crisis and recovery that imagines health as the end or beginning, as absence of action. After all, since its rise in the eighteenth century, the novel has persistently trained its readers to expect conflict and resolution, mysteries and solutions, a beginning that moves (but not too quickly) toward an end. The endings of eighteenth-century texts, such as Charlotte Lennox's *Female Quixote* (1752) and Tobias Smollett's *The Expedition of Humphrey Clinker* (1771), for example, spectacularly showcase cure from illness as the desired and achievable goal.

In this book, I consider the effort (and, as the medical advice warns, it takes effort) that goes into reading for health. I identify a model of reading that interprets health as more than a point of entry or of departure—as more than something to be "passively appreciated." The novels of Jane Austen, Charlotte Brontë, Harriet Martineau, Charles Dickens, and Elizabeth Gaskell—novels that prominently feature invalids and their doctors, contagions and fevers, sicknesses and cures—provide lessons not only in how to be healthy but also in how to read for health. Whereas a study such as Haley's offers insight into the former, this book seeks to broaden our understanding of the latter by exploring the difficulty of replacing the familiar narrative arc of prelude, crisis, and cure (which I refer to as *therapeutic*) with one centered on more-static models of maintenance and prevention (what I am calling *hygienic*). The novelists and medical advisers featured in the following chapters demonstrate that health has a narrative of its own, one that complements even as it complicates the linearity of the disease-cure model. Through cautionary tales and secondary narratives and characters, the writers I study provide strategies for reading others and the environment for hygienic purposes. Reading for health's narrative challenges our sense of order and temporality, setting and metaphor, point of view and voice. It means reading for what has largely remained unread.

Physicians have long registered their concern about society's passive appreciation of health. In *The Code of Health and Longevity* (1807), Sir John Sinclair laments, "People seldom attend to their health till it be too late. They scarcely ever think of it till they are seriously impaired."[19] The year before, Thomas Beddoes supposed in his *Manual of Health* (1806) that "could you but once lead the public to suspect that health may be SOMEWHAT OF AN ACCOMPLISHMENT, they would then, I think, cultivate it uninterruptedly without grudging, and not dismiss it as shortly as they can, like an importunate creditor."[20] By the end of the century, James Hinton was still warning readers in *Thoughts on Health* (1871), "The time for unconscious fulfillment of the laws of health has practically past. We must either know or suffer."[21] These criticisms recur in numerous medical and nonmedical texts throughout the eighteenth and nineteenth centuries, a time during which handbooks such as these rose in popularity and accessibility. The prevalence of so many guides, pamphlets, and memoirs that warn readers about their ignorance and their inability to attend properly to health attests to a cultural desire—compulsion, even—to read and write about, and to imagine, health.[22] The mass of material during this period also registers an epistemological anxiety about the possibility of ever truly knowing health. Victorian surgeon John Milner Fothergill captures this concern when he exclaims in the introduction to *The Maintenance of Health* (1874), "Health! What is it? And how is it maintained?"[23] Health is both something we can assert emphatically ("Health!") and something that remains a mystery ("What is it?").

An entire industry was dedicated (and still is) to answering Fothergill's questions and to helping readers solve the mystery of health, which was often imagined in vague yet alluring terms. Fothergill claims that health is the "balance betwixt the various parts of the organism" (1), whereas Hinton declares that it involves being in "harmony with the ceaseless activities of nature" (*Thoughts,* 333). Such a view of health explains why it is easy to ignore and why it seems to fail as a model for narrative. Health is or should be unremarkable: "[N]o man is truly healthy," Hinton claims, "who is thinking about his health" (332). We might think here of Aristotle's conception of tragedy; his emphasis on catastrophe and the consequent catharsis (purification) as offering an early articulation of this critical investment in crisis and cure. But even Hinton's definition of health's congruence signifies its narrative potential: health "exists in ceaseless adaptation to all the infinite variety of nature—ever the same, yet ever new. . . . Health knows no *monotony*" (333, emphasis added). Such claims allow us to interpret health as largely a process, a movement, or an act of loss or gain—in short, as narrative.

The desire to foreground health's narratability—to make it legible—has been central to medical advice since antiquity. As Greek physician and philosopher Galen explains, health is part one of a two-part story: "Since, both in importance and in time, health precedes disease, so we ought to consider first how health may be preserved, and then how one may best cure disease."[24] P. N. Singer notes in the introduction to his translation of *Galen: Selected Works* that doctors, such as Galen, were part of the Roman elites' "daily entourage" and that health was, since at least "Hippocratic times[,] . . . something which involve[d] certain types of constant, daily practice for its maintenance."[25] The advice Galen and subsequent medical writers offer distinguishes between health and disease, between the "daily practice" and the temporary treatment. "Whereas the science concerned with the human body is one," Galen notes, "its foremost and largest subdivisions are two: one of these is called hygiene, the other therapeutics, differing in their respective functions, the former being concerned to maintain, the latter to modify, the condition of the body."[26]

Galen's demarcation between hygiene and therapeutics, as well as the format of his medical advice, persisted with surprisingly little alteration—given the changes in medical knowledge—well into the nineteenth century. The concern that medical writers express about their readers' inability to recognize health did not originate in the nineteenth century, and it certainly did not end there; but the availability of written material on the subject, the developments in medicine, and the vastness of the reading public converged during the nineteenth century to make it a period of intense debate about health, particularly in terms of the two categories of medicine—hygiene and therapeutics—that Galen identified. For although these categories are interrelated, advice books by medical professionals and laypersons alike often emphasize one over the other. William Strange, for example, wrote predominantly on the restoration of health,[27] or therapeutics, whereas Sinclair focused on hygiene, organizing the sixth edition of his *Code of Health and Longevity* (1844) "under three general heads:—on the means, 1. Of preserving health, 2. Of prolonging life, and 3. Of curing or alleviating disease" (3). The first two headings (preserving and prolonging) fall under the umbrella term of maintenance (hygiene), while the third is dedicated to therapeutics. Sinclair employs this formula in part because he was not an expert on cure. But more than that, he (like many other writers) was aware of or concerned about the notion that readers think too much about cure. The reading public, among whom Sinclair includes medical professionals, needs to attend more to the story of health than to that of disease. Thus, while I am interested in the narrative structures that make health legible—a text to be read and followed—I want to demonstrate how these structures and how reading "hygienically" function as a form of resistance to dominant modes of thought, particularly the curative or "therapeutic" ethos, which seeks closure and a definitive end.

I attend to these issues not to suggest that disease and closure are unimportant or that the ability to find solutions for them is unworthy of our attention. Getting sick is terrifying, and it was particularly so during the period before germ theory was fully accepted, when a simple cut could lead to a life-threatening infection or a drink of water could unleash a deadly epidemic. But wherever possible, avoiding illness in the first place is safer than relying on treatment. Sinclair was not a medical man, but his work offers a plan for health based on his extensive reading (it summarizes several popular medical guides) and his own experience. Influenced by Galenic theories of medicine that tout the importance of moderation in diet and exercise, he counsels readers, "The foundation should be laid early; the plan or system should begin in youth, and ought afterwards resolutely to be persevered in" (1844 *Code,* 10), while acknowledging that the perseverance (or narrative "drive") perhaps more than the plan (or "plot") is what readers seem to resist. He criticizes those who "represent hygeian rules as troublesome; and account all persons as miserable, who live according to any regular system," promising instead that "pleasure," or what we might call narrative fulfillment, comes from developing "habits" of health (14).

Novelists such as Austen, Brontë, Martineau, Dickens, and Gaskell not only thematize and satirize the details of these "plans" (recall Mr. Woodhouse's concern about wedding cake in *Emma*) but also incorporate the notion of perseverance and daily practice into the very form of their narratives. Jane Austen's *Sense and Sensibility* and Charlotte Brontë's *Jane Eyre,* for example, may feature therapeutics as integral to the advancement of their heroines' plots and seem almost wholly organized around the crisis (or multiple crises) they must endure, but these plots are governed equally, if not so obviously, by a hygienic model of narrative. They reflect a desire to maintain rather than simply treat, to prevent rather than cure. In these narratives, the ostensibly dilatory state of health intersects with and subsumes the teleological impulse of disease. These novels teach us an alternative rhythm of reading, one that operates outside the comfort of cure and the allure of disease and invites readers to revise their expectations about character development (bildungsroman), the narrator's authority (omniscience and reliability), narrative closure (essential to marriage plots), and the metaphorical language associated with these structural elements, which align with the critical investment in illness.

Although determining what people knew about health and whether or not they were accurate in that knowledge is of interest in this book,[28] I am more concerned with identifying the ways authors write about such topics—the narrative strategies used by novelists and medical writers when trying to preserve, promote, and define health and the reading practices these strategies invite or impose.[29] *Reading for Health*'s focus on the narrative of health has been shaped, as the title implies, by Peter Brooks's *Reading for the Plot* (1984) and D. A. Miller's *Narrative and its Discontents* (1989), as both critics examine the reader's and the narrative's relationship to beginnings and ends and to the traditional narrative of crisis and recovery.[30] Brooks challenges "the static models" of narrative developed by formalists, because they fail to account for "reading narrative as a dynamic operation." He uses metaphors such as "motor" and "engine" to explain the type of movement that occurs in narrative, and he couples this model with a Freudian understanding of psychic mobility, suggesting that desire for the end (the death instinct) initiates the narrative and drives the plot. As he explains it, "Narrative desire is ultimately, inexorably, desire *for* the end."[31] But even as Brooks asserts the death drive as narrative's primary force, he calls on the language of medicine to describe this narrative event. In his examination of *Great Expectations* (1860–61), for example, he argues, "At the end [of the novel] we have the impression of a life that has outlived plot, renounced plot, been *cured* of it: life that is left over." "Plot," he suggests, "comes to resemble a diseased, fevered state of the organism."[32] Medical rhetoric, particularly the language associated with crisis and recovery, seeps naturally into theories of narrative action.

For Miller, "narratability" is "the instance of disequilibrium, suspense, and general insufficiency from which a given narrative appears to arise."[33] Miller offers Mary and Henry Crawford from Austen's *Mansfield Park* (1814) as examples, noting that both characters defer textual closure—Henry through his flirtatious behavior and refusal to commit to marriage and Mary through discourse, her "perpetual promise and deferral of knowledge and right nomination." Miller highlights these two characters because, for Austen, narratability "coincides with what the novelist strongly disapproves of (waywardness, flirtation) and . . . closure is associated with her most important official values (settlement, moral insight, and judgment)." These nonnarratable, or "healthy," behaviors are, for Miller and others, what the novel (and the novel reader) seeks to achieve.

In another example, Miller explains that we know Emma Woodhouse has been "cured" when she begins to think of herself in terms of her "blindness" and "blunders," when her language shifts from self-absorbed to self-aware.[34] Both Miller and Brooks call on the language of health (cure and recovery) to construct their theories.[35] In doing so, they highlight the notion that traditional narratives are marked by the drive toward cure, toward expelling that which is undesirable or diseased.

But just as a story in which everyone is healthy and happy is no story at all, neither is one in which all the characters are constantly sick. We need, as Brooks might argue, the detours that move us between these two states and keep us slightly off-balance. Miriam Bailin challenges the traditional view that health and cure are fiction's desired and necessary end, arguing in her study on the Victorian sickroom that "[t]he conventional pattern of ordeal and recovery takes on its particularly Victorian emphasis in the location of the desired condition of restored order and stability not in regained health but in a sustained condition of disability and quarantine."[36] Referring to Charlotte Brontë and Charles Dickens in particular, she goes on to argue that the "narrative cure for disorder is more often than not illness itself and the therapeutic situation constructed around it."[37] If, as Bailin proposes, the Victorian novel transforms illness into cure (narratively speaking), then I would like to suggest that it transforms health into action, into a kind of narrative crisis in itself. For, even as novels in the nineteenth century rely on the illness-cure model, another model, I argue, undergirds this traditional structure—one determined by the vagaries to be found within plots of health. Health is a precarious and subjective condition marked by uncertain chronologies, invented plots, and hopeful, vigilant characters. It insists on the simultaneous application of hindsight and foresight and provides writers narrative possibility rather than simply an ending, an ongoing drama rather than the absence or end of action.[38]

I turn briefly here to the great medical novel *Middlemarch*,[39] for although it is not central to my study, it was written by a novelist who, by 1872, had thoroughly absorbed the lessons of health that I identify in each of my chapters. Two moments from George Eliot's text exemplify how we might become more conscious of what it means to "read for health." At first, the scenes are so steeped in the language and metaphors of illness and therapeutics that it is difficult (more so than in the other texts I study) to read them "hygienically." Each episode involves the doctor-hero Tertius Lydgate, but neither features the doctor engaged in typical medical practice or relies on the clinical and scientific verisimilitude that is generally associated with Eliot's realism.[40] In the first, Eliot stages the scene of Nicholas Bulstrode's climactic expulsion from Middlemarch at a town meeting—significantly—about sanitary reform. The town's literal and figurative health is at stake, as the scandal surrounding the wealthy banker has the potential to infect all with whom he comes into contact. Mr. Hawley refuses to let Bulstrode comment on the town's sanitary concerns if Bulstrode is not himself free of taint, of scandal. Bulstrode cannot refute the allegation that he "was for many years engaged in nefarious practices, and that he won his fortune by dishonest procedures," and his body reveals as much—he becomes too weak to walk unassisted. Lydgate, though he realizes that any association with Bulstrode will harm his reputation, cannot refuse to see Bulstrode as his patient and must help: "What could he do?" (450). The narrator explains that Lydgate's "movement of resentful hatred was checked by his instinct of the Healer which thinks first of bringing rescue or relief to the sufferer" (449). At this point, the scene satisfies the requirements of the conventional crisis-cure narrative, underscored by the narrator's reference to Lydgate as "the Healer" (that is, one who cures). Bulstrode's narrative is in crisis, he becomes sick, and the doctor offers relief.

The action of this scene comes largely from the publicity of Bulstrode's misdeeds, but this moment also invokes a preventative impulse, inviting the reader to think of the past and future simultaneously. As any good physician knows, the doctor's job is not only to diagnose and cure but also to teach patients to avoid illness in the first place. In fact, if more of the latter occurred, less of the former would be needed. Bulstrode's illness and potential cure become a cautionary tale about the dangerous effects of past acts, while Lydgate's act of sympathy sets in motion his own tragic future. Had it not been for the doctor's instinct to offer the weak man his arm and lead him from the meeting, Lydgate would have been absorbed, at least temporarily, into the status quo. As a result of his sympathy, we begin to anticipate, along with Lydgate, the potential dangers of his actions—we begin, that is, to think "hygienically" in terms of prevention and preservation, becoming aware of that moment when Lydgate could have avoided future "dis-ease," and did not. The townsmen are similarly poised between a crisis-cure model, as they seek to exorcize their diseased part, and a hygienic one, enacting a quarantine to prevent further and future damage. Lydgate helps to remove Bulstrode, but "curing" Bulstrode's hypochondriasis or saving the town does not motivate his actions or drive the narrative. In fact, this type of "therapeutic" language, though not wrong in this case, is inadequate. The town and the narrative require Lydgate's sympathy, as "bitter" as it might be, more than they require any type of medical cure. And although this model of sympathy ultimately does not prevail, the impulse of health—of preservation and prevention—emerges momentarily as it pushes questions of moral and medical disease aside.

As the above example demonstrates, the shift I am tracing can be fleeting. As soon as it arises, it is subsumed by the prevailing discourse and metaphors of disease. We see this in a parallel moment when Dorothea posits a more intricate relationship between character transformation and health. Enlisting the kindly Reverend Camden Farebrother into a diagnostic assessment of Lydgate's condition, Dorothea tries to convince him that Lydgate is innocent of killing or purposely mistreating Raffles, the man who has exposed Bulstrode as a fraud. She asks Farebrother to consider Lydgate's character, to which he responds, "But my dear Mrs Casaubon . . . character is not cut in marble—it is not something solid and unalterable. It is something living and changing, and *may become* diseased as our bodies do" (454, emphasis added). Appropriating the language of medicine, interweaving therapeutics and hygiene, as Farebrother does, Dorothea responds in kind: "Then [character] *may be* rescued and healed" (454, emphasis added). Health, in this exchange, appears to be an end point, the result of sequestering Lydgate in a metaphorical sickroom and treating his illness—he will be healed. On the one hand, then, this scene seems to be (more so than the first example) a moment of crisis in need of cure. And to some extent it is, but we can see, too, that health and the actions one takes to preserve it are not simply about cures and ends. "The Healer" must think hygienically as well as therapeutically, and Dorothea's project, which does not work as she had hoped, registers a desire to do both: to institute a preventive model, something from which her own love plot may have benefited, and to hint at the possibility ("may become," "may be") of preservation rather than only of immediate cure. Health is a persistent, if often overlooked, force within narrative, a continuous and dynamic operation and, ultimately, a form of sustained compassion. As in the first episode, Eliot provides readers a model of social action that does not depend on the sickroom scene, so that thinking novelistically means turning to health rather than disease; it means opening our thinking to a wider range of possibilities and temporalities.

Reading for health involves, as medical advisers routinely assert, knowing what health is. Just as in the therapeutic model, wherein one must be sick to get cured, so too in the hygienic model one must recognize good health to maintain it. But as the novelists discussed in the following chapters demonstrate, and as the organization of this book suggests, defining health and maintaining it are interdependent narrative acts. One's ability to know what health is does not always precede one's attempts to maintain it. In fact, it is through the maintenance of health, particularly through acts of prevention, that we can know health, that it becomes a legible text that we become proficient in reading. We define our health, in other words, by the ways we interpret and modify our body's responses to, for example, the environment in which we live, the food we eat, the physical activity we exert, and the mental and physical hardships we endure.[41]

While the following chapters reflect an evolution of fictional form and medical practice during the nineteenth century, they do not aim to tell a linear or progressive history of either field. In fact, reading linearly and chronologically is, in part, what this book proposes to resist. I have organized the chapters into three parts to highlight the recursivity of health's narrative. Our attempts to manage health shape our definition of it, and the terms we use to define it govern how we manage it. Part 1 examines domestic health and personal conduct, whereas part 2 focuses on texts and characters that represent an unconventional view of health. Both parts alternate between chapters on prevention and chapters that seek to define health through maintenance. Part 3 departs from this model by turning to the realm of the professional (the physician and the physician's stand-in), who must become adept at reading for health. Such narrative competence is an essential instrument of medical practice and medical education.

Chapter 1 identifies prevention as the primary marker of the hygienic plot in Jane Austen's fiction; it competes with and overrides the more traditional therapeutic one. As I argue in this chapter, health, for Austen, has little to do with the pursuit or even the rejection of cure and everything to do with the absence of crisis. Although most novels ask us to invite risk, experience disease, and recover slowly, her fictions (*Sense and Sensibility* and *Mansfield Park,* in particular) move relentlessly to preempt disaster. "Recovery," then, is the work of ceaseless and anxious prevention. It means looking ahead to what might happen and looking back at what has been in order to manage current, healthful behavior. Austen's novels and the domestic medical guides discussed in this chapter—William Buchan's *Domestic Medicine* (1769) and Thomas Beddoes's *Hygeia*

(1802)—are equally intent on teaching their readers to think and to read as preventionists.

Jane Eyre, perhaps the best "reader" in this book, is a heroine whose preventionist instinct shapes her plot and, more importantly, her sense of self. Jane's autobiographical narration not only illustrates how to avoid the fates of other women in the novel (Helen Burns, Bertha Mason, and the would-be Mrs. St. John Rivers) but also depends on an active and aggressive assertion of what health means and her acute awareness that she must maintain it. She is not the "picture of health," as is Emma Woodhouse, but her narrative probes what it might mean to be the one who draws that picture. Chapter 2, therefore, focuses more directly on the strategies medical writers used to define the contours of health and on the narration and narrative desire that emerge around the twin objectives of identifying and preserving it. Health, as the medical dictionaries of the period suggest, is a recognizable condition as well as a range of conditions; it is capacious, rare, and always relative, unique to the individual but also generalizable to the community. *Jane Eyre*'s point of view and the "improvement" (marriage) plot to which it gives rise rely on the power and narrative authority that come from narrating one's health.

Part 2 is the rebellious sibling of part 1. While the two chapters in this section similarly disrupt the crisis-cure model of narrative, they also push back against the Austenian sense of prevention and complicate the Brontëan version of the healthy heroine. By first focusing on preventionist discourse of public health in the novels of Charles Dickens (chapter 3) and then on the definitional strategies that the invalid Harriet Martineau uses in her novel and memoir (chapter 4), I suggest that these novelists reflect a more combative relationship to the dominant health discourse of the period than do the novelists in part 1. Whereas Austen's novels advance and even refine the advice offered by preventionists who are concerned with domestic medicine, Dickens's *Little Dorrit* virtually rejects public health experts' opinions about the best policy for preventing epidemic disease. The sanitary reforms Dickens advocated in his speeches, his essays, and many of his novels (such as *Bleak House*) fade into the background in *Little Dorrit,* in which he features a competing and, for Dickens's occasional public health adviser Thomas Southwood Smith, dubious approach to the preservation of public health: quarantine. Rather than promote the kind of curative and preemptive action that is characteristic of the "sanitary method" and Austen's preventionist cautionary tales, Dickens turns to a more static and isolationist model of prevention that appears to court—even as it promises to obstruct—disease. Health depends on the risk associated with touch and on an almost willful refusal to look ahead to what might be or to learn from what has been.

If, as in the works of Dickens, we can achieve health through counterintuitive means, then the very definition of health is equally disputable. The chapters in this book represent health as a story we tell about ourselves within community and isolated from it. This story occasionally contradicts prevailing modes of thought about sanitary reform or, as in chapter 4, able-bodiedness. The figure of the invalid tests the limits of what health means. Is invalidism merely the opposite of health, or does it represent ideal health? I suggest that the works of Harriet Martineau and others redefine invalidism as a narrative stance rather than a social or physical condition exclusively marked as debility. The culture's interest in fitting invalidism into the larger discourse of health intersects with the invalid's desire to stake her claim in society. And it is through their privileged perspective *on* the health of others—a perspective figured as a form of health—that they assert their cultural and narrative authority. Like Charlotte Brontë's heroine, the invalids in this chapter resist a curative ethos in favor of a hygienic one; but instead of turning to prevention (avoidance), these characters embody a preservationist stance by claiming the fictional authority associated with omniscience. They are, in effect, health's narrators.

Chapter 5 and the afterword conclude this study by applying the lessons of hygienic reading explored in the first two parts to fictional and contemporary medical education. Here, I focus more particularly on the figure of the doctor as the one who most needs to learn from this alternative way of reading. For unlike the impatient readers Beddoes and others lament, the doctor stands out as lacking the requisite reading skills. In *Wives and Daughters* (1865), for example, Elizabeth Gaskell reimagines medical practice and the role of the "healer" as a version of domestic management that requires not only the management of families but also the management of their stories. She neither defies the doctor's professional privilege nor adopts it. Instead, she depicts the doctor's authority and his expertise as contingent on narrative competence—the ability, as Rita Charon and others define it in relationship to medical practice, to listen to, interpret, and ethically act on the stories of others.[42] This, Gaskell, tells us, is best taught and learned in the home and from the novel. I offer an extended close reading of *Wives and Daughters*, drawing together the various lessons of the previous chapters about domestic health, quarantines, healthy heroines, and invalidism. As I discuss in my afterword, this type of narrative competence is essential to medical education as a way of bridging the traditional divide between patients and their doctors. Contemporary work in the field of narrative medicine assumes, like Gaskell's novel, an integral relationship between storytelling and medical advice. By becoming attentive to the multiple ways that stories work—not only as symptoms of illness but also as strategies for sustaining health—doctors and patients can experience more humane and effective medical encounters. I am suggesting that such an approach to health and medicine is part of the legacy that medical advice and the nineteenth-century novel have left to their readers.

One

Domestication

Chapter One

Jane Austen's Plots of Prevention

In the second of eleven installments of *Hygeia* (1802–3),[1] Thomas Beddoes offers the following fictional dialogue between a woman and her doctor:

> "What is good against the head-ache, Doctor?"
>
> "Health, Madam."
>
> "Well, if you feel no interest about an old woman like me—Marianne there, you perceive, has been hacking all afternoon. Do tell her of some little thing, [*sic*] that is good against cough."
>
> "Health, Madam."
>
> "But are you resolved not to give a more satisfactory answer?" (14–15)

To make a case that prevention is more important than cure, Beddoes satirizes those who turn to their doctors for easy remedies—those bad readers who are too easily seduced by the drama of diagnosis, the action of treatment, and the closure of cure. In fact, Beddoes "explicitly declare[s] PREVENTION of mischief to be [his] exclusive objective," asking his readers in the second installment of *Hygeia* to "bear with [him] yet a few more months, before they give [him] up" (14) for the "makers of those books . . . which profess to distribute far and wide a capacity for discriminating diseases and applying remedies" (19). Health, conceived in this way, should not be about getting cured but about preventing illness in the first place. One does not become sick; rather, one loses the opportunity to stay well, and the woman's response to her beleaguered doctor suggests that such a concept was, if not difficult to accept, at least highly unsatisfactory. The fictional woman interprets the doctor's prescription ("Health, Madam") as a refusal to practice medicine, and while the adage "an ounce of prevention is worth a pound of cure" was common enough, it did not quite capture one's interest in the way that Widgeon's Purifying Pills did.[2]

Beddoes renders the distinction between taking "some little thing" and becoming a preventionist explicit in terms of its narrative aims: "Writings intended to warn against the destruction of health," he argues, "can hardly be confounded with such as pretend to teach people how to restore it. To direct a stranger how to traverse a slippery ground without injury is one thing. To instruct him how to set his leg should he break it, is quite another" ("Essay II" in *Hygeia,* 35). These instructions differ in terms of both their content and the form that they take—and to the reader addicted to the drama of broken legs, simply learning to traverse is not so immediately appealing. As Ginnie Smith explains in "Prescribing the Rules of Health: Self-Help and Advice in the Late Eighteenth Century," "Prevention . . . is and was barely newsworthy[,] being a passive or negative operation."[3] No statistics exist for the number of healthy citizens of a given period, so we cannot know if something has been prevented, we can only know when it has not. The great paradox at work in such narratives is that one can only write about prevention by showing what must be prevented—that is, showing what one wants to keep from happening. To grasp the significance of the warning, we must witness the destructiveness—the proverbial broken leg—that results from avoidable behavior.

Beddoes was certainly not alone in his struggle with this problem. In the highly popular *Domestic Medicine* (1769),[4] William

Buchan assumes that his readers will be disappointed in the dearth of "pompous prescriptions, and promised great cures" (vii) to be found in his manual, asserting that he "would much rather teach men how to avoid the necessity of using [pills and potions], than how they should be used" (viii). Physicians such as Buchan and Beddoes were acutely aware that the anxiety over disease (both moral and medical) and the satisfaction that comes with recovery made for a powerful narrative, one not easy for doctors promoting prevention to displace. As such, the problem was how to show what a narrative of prevention looks like. Readers of health manuals wanted to learn how to get well more than they wanted to learn how not to get sick.

The problems associated with narrating prevention hold true for the nineteenth-century novel. Indeed, the novel bears much of the responsibility for the seductiveness of the illness-cure trajectory, having trained its readers to expect conflicts that get resolved and longing that gets rewarded. Narrative arises when we get sick; closure happens because we get well.[5] Set during a period in which home health care guides were becoming more accessible than they had been in previous decades, Jane Austen's novels, though no stranger to the cure model of narrative, embrace this tension between stories that warn and stories that restore. Not only does Austen rely on her heroine's ailing body to govern, at least in part, how we read her story or how we read any story, but also she situates these crisis-cure moments (dangerous fevers and life-threatening falls) within and against narratives of prevention. Cure is, without a doubt, interesting, but as Austen's novels demonstrate, it is not the only way to tell a story.

Prevention offers a different way of thinking about any single event. It draws the past and the future into contact by asking us to look forward to a time when we will look backward in regret at our current moment, a moment when we were still (however precariously) healthy and could have done something to avoid disaster. Thus, at the same time that prevention turns our attention to the past, it conditions us to think in terms of the future and to imagine the foreknowledge that will help nip disease in the bud and offer a healthy, happy ending. Prevention often consists in taking action, such as getting inoculated, or, as Austen satirizes in the unfinished *Sanditon*, in doing silly things to perfectly healthy bodies: pulling teeth, taking emetics, applying leeches. But more often, prevention expects us *not* to do something (don't drink too much, don't touch that). However static this directive may seem, prevention's etymology—"to come before" (*præ* 'before' and *venīre* 'to come')—allows us to see the narrative opportunities, the intense activity, inherent to this way of thinking. The beforeness that defines prevention captures the imagined state of preserved health that turns plot into a constant caution not to "do" but to "not do" as we ought, redirecting narrative and readerly energy toward plots of averting, not anticipating—making us "patient readers."

Most health guides, like Austen's novels, focus their attention on middle-class family conduct and the role that parents play in educating their children and other subordinates. Buchan claims that he wanted to write *Domestic Medicine* in part because his patients needed a "plain directory for regulating their conduct" (xvi). Similarly, in a section in *Hygeia* entitled "Art of Preserving Health" ("Essay VI," 90), Beddoes advocates "practical instruction" for parents on "the structure of the human body." He even proposes public clinical and anatomical lectures for both men and women, the goal of which would be "to make fully sensible the mischief arising from systematic irregularity; from injudicious management after exposure to the inclemencies of weather, and from the other innumerable ordinary errors of individual conduct. [The lectures] must explain the origin and conduct, much more minutely than the treatment of disease" (91). Beddoes sounds like a novelist, highlighting not only "irregularity" and "injudiciousness" but also "ordinary errors" that shape character action or, as he puts it, "individual conduct." By focusing his readers' attention on the body and health as it relates to management, rather than to treatment, Beddoes enacts a subtle but important shift from cure to prevention. Certainly, therapeutics depend heavily on the compliant patient, but both physicians assume that patients are almost too willing at times to follow doctor's orders when it comes to cures. Buchan and Beddoes offer a prescription for health, as they encourage—even *require*—individuals to observe the vicissitudes of their own and others' bodies in a way that conforms to their expert opinion. As Beddoes asserts, "There is nothing [mankind is] so slow in learning, as how to direct their foresight, and portion out their cares properly."[6] For Austen, such foresight translates into learning to "do as one ought." Indeed, a preventionist ethic assumes and even creates the "ought" with which Austen's novels are, as critics have noted, so concerned and consumed.[7]

The first line of prevention is always a narrative one, and cautionary tales provide both the content and the formal structure of preventionist thinking. These stories assume a past (someone else's) of disease, debility, and even death. These stories about what has been and what might be thus feature "characters" who behave imprudently and suffer greatly because of it. In a section on the "consumptive disposition" in "Essay VII," for example, Beddoes transcribes a story written by one of his patients, Louisa, as a warning to his readers about the dangers of consumption or tuberculosis. She begins quite simply: "Our family was large." She goes on, as the narrator of a domestic novel might, to describe this family: "There were twelve of us in all, eight sisters and four brothers. I do not reckon three others, [*sic*] that died in their infancy." Louisa reaches back into her family history, noting that with the exception of her grandfather's gout, "no hereditary disorder had appeared on either side." The family's problems developed as a result of her father's "ambitio[n] that his sons should shine" and that his daughters should "have more information than in general falls to the share of women" (10). Initially, his attentiveness appeared progressive, but as his ambition turned into vanity and degenerated into neglect, the children suffered. Instead of merely describing her symptoms or speculating about proximate causes for her consumption, Louisa offers a narrative of what happens to the children of well-meaning but vain and ignorant parents. They "grow up to be the veriest of wretches," because in such a household, "health [is] never a constant, and seldom an occasional, concern" (12). In Louisa's tale, domestic management—a basic understanding of what constitutes a proper diet, exercise, climate, and leisure activities—is the source of prevention, for only a well-run household, we surmise, produces healthy, happy children.

For this reason, Buchan and Beddoes both begin their narratives before the problems, stresses, and dangers that come from living in the world infect the healthy body. In the first chapter of his *Domestic Medicine,* Buchan offers an earlier version of the cautionary tale Beddoes's Louisa tells. Buchan highlights the importance of our pasts—our childhoods—to our future health: "The better to trace diseases from their original causes, we shall take a view of the common treatment of mankind in the state of infancy. In this period of our lives, the foundations of a good or bad constitution are laid" (1). Buchan uses an architectural metaphor to emphasize the relationship between the health of the home and the health of the individual. Beddoes offers a similar metaphor in *Hygeia* to describe the importance of this originary moment and the consequences of domestic management. He notes that bad childrearing is akin to "rearing an edifice without tie or foundation, in the face of a tempestuous sky!" ("Essay I," 26). The value of this metaphor relies on the reader's awareness—and fear—of shaky structures. The family, then, is like a house, and raising either without proper forethought and guidance will lead to its future destruction.[8]

The lessons for genuinely healthy conduct, if there are to be any, must come from the home. Parents must be taught, through the stories their doctors tell them, how to instill these lessons in their children. For this reason, the works of Beddoes and Buchan, which focus on what parents should do for their as-yet-uninjured children, differ from earlier eighteenth-century manuals that address their advice to sick adults.[9] To be sure, both doctors' manuals offer directives to the intemperate or consumptive adult individual, but they do so only after establishing the importance of parental care in laying a foundation for future health. In *Domestic Medicine,* Buchan anticipates Austen and numerous Victorian novelists after her by blaming mothers for their ignorance and fathers for their lack of interest. He laments "that more care is not bestowed in teaching the proper management of children to those whom nature has designed for mothers" (2) and that the gentleman father is more interested in the management of his dogs and horses than his own child, "the heir of his fortunes, and the future hope of his country" (3). And these are the healthy parents. If the parents are diseased to begin with, their chances of raising healthy children diminish greatly. Although Buchan blames both parents, suggesting, "No person who labours under any incurable malady ought to marry" (5), the health of the child falls primarily to the mother. Taking a cue from Jean-Jacques Rousseau's *Emile,* Buchan warns, "A delicate female, brought up within doors, an utter stranger to exercise and open air, who lives on tea and other slops, may bring a child into the world, but it will hardly be fit to live" (4). Buchan argues that, in some instances, the best way to prevent disease or debility is to prevent life in the first place.

Beddoes does not go as far as Buchan, but he similarly focuses his attention on what parents do wrong. Beddoes's advice acts as a warning and a plea; for the manual, he claims, will help these parents "equip [their] children, as they advance to that age when they must be left to their own guidance, with the most precise instructions respecting the hazards they will soon have to encounter" ("Essay I" in *Hygeia,* 15). *Hygeia* demonstrates over the next thousand pages what Austen takes only a few hundred to show: how a mismanaged household produces debilitated children who grow up to be wretched adults. Bad diet, lack of exercise, poor schooling conditions, and intemperance—all the stuff of which novels are made—are just some of the "hazards" children suffer when left "to their own guidance." The more pernicious activities of masturbation, shopping, and novel reading similarly matter less as moral vice than as detrimental to the medical health of the household.

But such medical advice is as much about the physical conditions of the body as it is about the moral condition of the soul. The full subtitle of Beddoes's collection, *Essays Moral and Medical, on the Causes Affecting the Personal State of Our Middling and Affluent Classes,* articulates this connection, and in his first essay he instructs his readers that "[t]o form a moral *sense* . . . is not more practicable in itself, than to form a *sense* for health, or for happiness, which latter must be, in great measure, composed of the sense of health" (84). Beddoes conflates the moral and the medical to construct a comprehensive story of middle-class conduct, and he demands that his readers become moral managers of their own bodies and the bodies of those around them, particularly their children. To emphasize his point, he ends his first essay by asking his readers to imagine their own child, "[t]hat being, whose happy smiles thou art now watching," crying out in the future, "Ah! had not the affection of my parents been as blind as it was strong, never should I have been the wretch I am" (92). Beddoes does not simply explain causes to his readers so that they can avoid their effects; he creates characters we recognize from the fictional narratives that nineteenth-century novelists reverted to time and again. We hear traces of the story of the fallen woman and the profligate son, whose demises were initiated by ignorant parents. Beddoes offers this ominous ventriloquizing of the reader's child as a "wretch" in the future to suggest that parental responsibility is the key to familial health and happiness. As the last sentence of his first essay, this remark is quite a cliffhanger. What parent, especially one with strong affections, would not look out anxiously for the next essay, while keeping a more vigilant eye on his or her child and anticipating fresh dangers?

PREVENTION AND CURE IN *Sense and Sensibility*

Austen's novels, which are also sympathetic to the relationship between the moral and the medical, do not allow for such a tidy elision between the two. Like the physicians, Austen targets negligent parents—though with a decidedly sharper wit and a more nuanced approach. Bad domestic managers are bad preventionists. In *Sense and Sensibility* (1811),[10] Austen depicts the type of affectionately neglectful parent to whom Beddoes might be addressing his essays. Nobody doubts Mrs. Dashwood's maternal affection, but we all recognize that she is more than a little "blind" to the truth of her middle daughter's affair. The plot that unfolds, Beddoes might suggest, is a result of domestic mismanagement and a lack of foresight. From the start, *Sense and Sensibility* functions not so much as a manual of what to do or even of how to recover from what has been; rather, its structure relies heavily on the tension between preventing what might happen and curing what has happened. As such, Austen organizes her first novel around the discursive parallels between cure and prevention, between the cautionary wretch, Marianne Dashwood, and her more vigilant, older sister, Elinor. For example, during Marianne's initial encounter with her would-be lover, Willoughby, when she twists her ankle, all propriety is lost in the face of physical harm. Willoughby, a complete stranger, must carry Marianne through the rain. Although her embarrassment prohibits Marianne from fully examining him, "his person and air were equal to what her fancy had ever drawn for the hero of her favourite story" (38), a story that soon becomes all too real. Willoughby's constant overtures eventually lead everyone except Elinor to assume that the couple is engaged. When Willoughby takes his leave of Barton, Elinor's foresight directs her to urge Mrs. Dashwood into proper conduct and to ask Marianne whether she and Willoughby have a formal understanding. Mrs. Dashwood's refusal should remind us of those bad parents that Buchan and Beddoes describe. The narrator tells us that "common sense, common care, common prudence, were all sunk in Mrs. Dashwood's romantic delicacy" (74).

Like her mother, Marianne ignores "foresight" in favor of romance. She would rather be a wretch than have no story at all. To this end, Marianne refuses to eat, finds it "very inexcusable" to sleep, and develops a "head-ache" in response to her lover's departure. This unchecked grief initiates her decline and turns into the type of narrative that requires either cure or death at its end. But before she is fully sunk, Marianne embraces her grief. Buchan explains that while grief is natural, to embrace it is a potentially dangerous precursor to wretchedness. In "On Grief" in *Domestic Medicine,* Buchan offers guidance for preventing the physical decline that attends this "Passion of the Mind." When in a state of grief, he suggests, we should "turn the attention frequently to new objects. Examine them for some time. When the mind begins to recoil, shift the scene. By this means a constant succession of new ideas may be kept up, till the disagreeable ones entirely disappear." "Indolence," he warns, "nourishes grief."[11] Austen initially presents Marianne's behavior as comical—we are meant to laugh at the deliberateness of Marianne's romantic symptoms. But beneath the absurdity of her behavior lurk the seriousness of Buchan's warning and the potentially tragic outcome of Marianne's conduct. The narrator tells us that Marianne plays Willoughby's favorite songs and "read[s] nothing but what they had been used to read together." In short, she does the opposite of what the manuals recommend. "This nourishment of grief," we are told, "was applied [by Marianne] every day" (73). Nourishment generally has a positive association; we might think of hearty food or mother's milk or any number of domestic terms that invoke home, health, and care, which contrast with Marianne's rejection of such things. Buchan's use of the term *nourish* thus hints at the domestic aspects of indolence and grief. Indolence occurs in the home and therefore comes under the purview of domestic management.

Austen adopts this sense of indolence but undercuts the danger we have learned to read into it from Buchan by recasting nourishment as the act of a silly young girl. Like Buchan, Austen applies the term to something that should not be nourished. An important difference between their usages is the agent of the action. For Buchan, indolence does the nourishing. For Austen, Marianne does. Buchan recommends that the grieved reader replace the sad story that has resulted in her current condition with a "new," more agreeable one. Instead of following this model, Marianne cares for and nurtures her grief, deliberately allowing it to grow. Yet rather than simply condemning Marianne for, in some sense, failing to follow Buchan's advice, Austen depicts her actions as necessary to the plot. Had Marianne properly prevented her grief—indeed, stopped it from growing—her narrative might well have stopped there. Instead, this grief becomes the first in a series of presumably preventable yet highly desirable and narratable episodes that propel the story and must, we expect, move us toward cure.[12] Marianne's resistance to prevention nourishes the narrative of cure, and the struggle between these two narratives—not simply the presence of crisis—energizes the novel.

But lest this sound like a familiar version of the crisis-cure plot, Austen's anatomy of wretchedness offers an alternative style of grief management through the parallel plot of Elinor, the novel's chief preventionist. During Edward Ferrars's final visit to Barton in the first half of the novel, Elinor senses a difference in his treatment of her. She does not, at this point in the novel, know that Edward is engaged to Lucy Steele, but the changes she detects are enough to cause her grief. Instead of indulging her grief, however, Elinor becomes "determin[ed] to subdue it, and to prevent herself from appearing to suffer." "She did not," the narrator tells us, "adopt the method so judiciously employed by Marianne, on a similar occasion, to augment and fix her sorrow, by seeking silence, solitude and idleness." Elinor is not invested in the romance of cure in the way that Marianne is; rather, Elinor "[sits] down to her drawing-table . . . [and] busily employ[s] herself the whole day" (90). So far, Elinor engages in recommended behavior, and Austen appears to be adhering to Buchan's guidance. But the narrator explains, "[Elinor's] thoughts could not be chained elsewhere . . . these thoughts must be before her, must force her attention" (91). Instead of complying entirely with popular advice for managing grief—that is, thinking of "new ideas"—Elinor allows her mind to reminisce freely on memories and indulge in fantasies built on her love for Edward (91). Despite Buchan's claims to the contrary, this type of attentiveness to one's grief—the presentness of one's thoughts—proves not only unavoidable, even by the best preventionists, but also beneficial. Upon the Steeles' departure, just after Lucy tells Elinor of her engagement to Edward, Elinor finds herself "at liberty to think and be wretched" (114). Only in private can Elinor accept and acknowledge, and therefore manage, her wretchedness. Elinor's failure to look for new ideas seems a rejection of preventative advice, but her actions invoke a sense of privacy and reflect an understanding of the relationship between the past and the present that prevention deems important.

At the same time that Elinor attempts to protect herself from decline, she must keep Marianne from becoming the heroine of a cautionary tale. From jokes about the intensity of Marianne's feelings to scoldings about accepting inappropriate gifts from Willoughby, Elinor holds firm to the spirit of prevention, lovingly coaxing Marianne into healthier conduct. In London, after witnessing Marianne's persistent, futile, and improper attempts to correspond with Willoughby, Elinor invokes the specter of the precautionary "wretch" by writing to her mother, in order, the narrator says, "to awake[n] her fears for the health of Marianne" and get her "to procure those inquiries which had so long been delayed" (145). Such inquiries, Elinor hopes, will force Marianne to acknowledge that she has been participating in a romantic fantasy and therefore save her from becoming the tragic heroine in a love story of her own making. Elinor thus imagines the story that could be—indeed, the story that we know has already been written by Austen—to manage its outcome.

Austen pits Elinor's plot of prevention against Marianne's plot of crisis and cure. For as the manuals suggest, the only way to render the narrative of prevention intelligible is by framing it in relation to—or even as a form of—cure. By the time Austen wrote *Mansfield Park,* she had ceased to rely on such framing and focused all the narrative's energies on prevention. But in this early novel, we experience a clear or at least clearer demarcation between the curative model and the preventative one. When Marianne finally learns of Willoughby's engagement to another woman, she becomes the self-described wretch that Beddoes portends and that Elinor fears. After Willoughby rebuffs Marianne at a London party and returns her letters, Marianne resists Elinor's remonstrance to maintain her composure. She cries out, "I care not who knows I am wretched. . . . I must feel—I must be wretched" (160). Austen invokes the wretched child, the figure on whom preventative medicine relies and for whom it laments, but she revises the meaning of the child's cries. Marianne embraces her wretchedness just as she nourished her grief, as if it were precisely what she was waiting for all along. Despite Elinor's best attempts to prevent Marianne's wretchedness (a state we already know she has experienced herself), Marianne claims she "must feel" and "must be" the wretch. In some respects, Elinor's attempt to teach Mrs. Dashwood the methods of prevention is an attempt to regulate how Marianne conducts herself and, thus, what Marianne signifies in the novel.

But while Elinor attempts to prevent Marianne's wretchedness, and while her parallel plot marks the difference between prevention and cure, the stories of two other wretched women perform, both thematically and structurally, the work of prevention. All of Austen's novels have, to varying degrees, embedded narratives that function as warnings—stories that "come before" (*prœ venīre*) the main narrative. In *Sense and Sensibility*, the stories of Eliza Brandon and her daughter, Eliza Williams, precede Marianne's and Elinor's plots of wretchedness.[13] The flannel-waistcoated Colonel Brandon, the novel's other preventionist, introduces these stories, believing that the story of the younger Eliza will be useful to Marianne. He begins his narrative by referring to events that precede the novel's beginning, as well as others that occurred earlier within the time frame of the novel but were never narrated. He tells Elinor about his love for Eliza Brandon, who he claims resembles "in some measure" Marianne (173). He speaks of her coerced marriage to his brother, the subsequent divorce, and her tragic decline into disrepute. He describes how he found her in a sponging house, a "melancholy and sickly figure" in the last stage of consumption.[14] This story of lost love precedes the story more relevant to Marianne's case: Willoughby's affair with Eliza Williams and the pregnancy that resulted from it. Austen delays this information to give the reader the time and reason to appreciate Colonel Brandon's attraction to Marianne and to anticipate Marianne's eventual acceptance of him as a husband. But for the purpose of prevention, this part of the story is also important in that it rehearses the deadly consequences of improper conduct by one who was so "blooming" and "healthful"—it is a story that just did not have to be (175).

The younger Eliza's story echoes a portion of her mother's, beginning, as the wretch's narrative must, with domestic mismanagement and parental neglect. At three years old, Eliza came under the guardianship of Colonel Brandon, who, having "no family, no home," placed Eliza at school, with a "very respectable woman" (176). Unfortunately, respectability was not quite the guard against wretchedness that the Colonel had hoped—if only he had paid attention to the first Eliza Brandon's story. At sixteen, Eliza Williams visited Bath with a young friend and her "well-meaning, but not quick-sighted father" (176)—yet another ignorant parent. Under such care, the impressionable and orphaned young Eliza was easily ruined and left by Willoughby. When the Colonel tells Elinor this story, Eliza has been hidden away in the country with her bastard child.

Although we can read both of the Eliza stories as cautionary tales of what Marianne might have become, Colonel Brandon does not exactly mean for Marianne to draw parallels between herself and the Elizas, despite the resemblance. Rather, he presents their stories to Elinor as examples of how well Marianne behaved, comparatively speaking. She has the potential for prevention after all. Brandon hopes that she will "turn with gratitude towards her own condition, when she compares it with that of [his] poor Eliza, when she considers the wretched and hopeless situation of this poor girl." Marianne's sufferings "proceed from no misconduct, and can bring no disgrace" (177). Although Austen condemns Marianne's behavior more than the colonel does, she depicts Marianne's wretchedness and misconduct as proceeding from domestic mismanagement and from a crucial failure of what Beddoes might refer to as her "health sense." A "[c]onsciousness of health," Beddoes explains, "will become just as much a source of pleasure as the consciousness of virtue."[15] The novel works toward helping Marianne reach this level of awareness and health—or, more specifically, it works toward helping the reader see how Marianne develops this sense.

Colonel Brandon aids the reader by pointing out that although Marianne has been saved from the moral fate of the Elizas, she remains in danger of suffering the same physical consequence and thus has not quite achieved that balance between virtue and health. Part of the tragedy for Colonel Brandon is that the previously healthy girl he loves has become melancholy and sickly. Eliza's social decline, we are led to believe, initiates a physical one. One must have the sense to know that improper attachments are both physically and morally unhealthy. The Elizas are Austen's version of the cautionary wretch, but they do not entirely work in the way we might think they should, for even after hearing their sad tales from Elinor, Marianne continues to neglect her health. Her "violent" cold comes on the heels of two long walks in the "longest and wettest" part of the grass, after which she "[sat] around in her wet shoes and stockings" (259). Her cold turns into an almost fatal fever, which begins to resemble the physical decline we imagine having preceded Eliza Brandon's consumption. The Eliza stories reach back into the past as a means of predicting the future and of developing not so much Marianne's but the reader's narrative foresight.

Before either Marianne or Elinor can find happiness in marriage, Marianne must emerge from her fever with a clearer moral and health sense. Once out of physical danger, Marianne expresses her wish that Willoughby not suffer too much. In response to this,

Elinor asks, "Do you compare your conduct with his?" "No," Marianne replies, "I compare it with what it ought to have been; I compare it with yours" (293). This comparison is what Austen has been encouraging her readers to make all along. But although we can read Marianne's contrite "what it ought to have been" as a reference or comparison to Elinor, we can also read it in terms of prevention. A semicolon interrupts Marianne's claim that she should have compared her behavior to her sister's. Certainly, the syntax of the sentence asks us to read the pause between "ought to have been" and "yours" as Marianne's recognition of Elinor's superior—healthier—conduct. However, we might also read the semicolon as an "and," separating the two claims. For underneath the comparison between Marianne and her sister lies the more tragic one between Marianne and the truly wretched women who haunt this novel, the two Elizas. The reader, if not Marianne, recognizes that through almost no will of her own, Marianne has survived an ordeal that two women before her did not—theirs ought to have been her fate, too.

PREVENTION AS NARRATIVE: *Mansfield Park*

In *Sense and Sensibility,* Austen articulates the difference between cure and prevention—between "happily ever after" and what "ought to have been"—through the parallel plots of Marianne and Elinor and through the cautionary tale of the two Elizas. In her "mature" work, Austen embeds prevention into the deep structure of her narrative, and within a single and singular heroine, Fanny Price. *Mansfield Park* (1814),[16] more than *Sense and Sensibility,* is interested in exposing root causes as a means of avoiding future effects; it is a novel about rendering the imagined story of what "comes before" in order to prevent what could be. Not that there is nothing to cure in *Mansfield Park:* Fanny's mother hopes she will become "materially better for change of air" (11); Tom Bertram's drinking causes him to suffer a life-threatening fever; Mary Crawford's cynical views of marriage prompt her aunt to worry that Mary is too much like her brother, Henry, and to claim that "Mansfield shall cure [them] both." "Stay with us," Mrs. Grant advises, "and we will cure you" (40). But for all its talk of cures, *Mansfield Park* is not fully governed by cure's narrative properties. In fact, Austen offers and then rejects at least two cure plots: the one that Mary Crawford imagines for her brother to which we shall return, and the more significant one that we as readers imagine for Fanny, one in which the "puny" and invisible heroine will grow into the belle of the ball. For although Fanny does become, as Lionel Trilling points out, "taller, prettier, and more energetic,"[17] she does not improve as much as or in the way that we might expect of a heroine. Fanny never achieves the physical or mental strength of an Anne Elliot or an Emma Woodhouse, as generations of cure-minded readers and critics have observed.[18]

That is not, however, because this is a bad novel: it is because Austen is doing something different here, teaching us something else. She is instructing us not to improve but to sustain, not to look ahead to the "multiple possible outcomes of a single moment in history"[19] or to forget a traumatic past,[20] but to look forward and backward simultaneously, not to cure but to prevent. For prevention in *Mansfield Park,* as in the medical discourse, is built on the tension between longing and fearing, between an idealized past and a threatening future; Fanny Price, with her wretched past and her vigilance about the future, is ideally suited for this preventionist project of protecting characters, revealing plots, and inoculating readers.

In a pivotal scene of prevention, one that critics like Marilyn Butler describe as the "ideological key to the novel" (224), Fanny sits on the sidelines, worrying as usual and cautioning her cousin Maria Bertram "not to slip" into the ha-ha. We witness more than just disapproval of Maria—who, after all, does not slip, though she will get seriously hurt. Fanny fails to stop the engaged Maria from following Henry Crawford instead of waiting for her fiancé. Nevertheless, she does succeed in the other intervention of this scene: keeping Edmund from following Mary Crawford into disaster. We mistake the larger purposes of the novel, however, if we read only for Fanny's incidental successes and failures. She cannot prevent Maria's "fall"; she cannot entirely preserve the Bertram estate; she barely manages to save Edmund. What she does do effectively is restore prevention as the source of good, for both characters and readers. For prevention proceeds along both of these tracks in the novel: not only must Edmund be preserved, but also readers must be educated. If for Edmund prevention is a course of abstinence—in which he must not marry Mary Crawford—so, too, is it for readers, who must retrain themselves in the value of delay, learning not to "slip." Just as Edward holds back, so must we, and it is through both its characters' travails and its temporal displacements that the novel teaches the art of prevention. And as with *Sense and Sensibility*, this lesson begins at home.

The Bertrams and the Prices, though separated by class and geography, are united in their lack of "health sense." Both households are home to spoiled, misbehaving children and distracted, disengaged parents, and the narrator describes the mismanagement of both: Portsmouth is a "scene of mismanagement" (324) just as Mansfield Park is a place of "grievous mismanagement" (382). Initially, the Prices are more easy to condemn, as the narrator criticizes them in the first chapter for being out of control and bursting at the seams, while allowing the Bertrams, particularly Sir Thomas, to sound like careful domestic managers. Mrs. Price must reconcile with her sisters after an eleven-year rift because as she "prepar[es] for her ninth lying-in," she fears for "the future maintenance" of the eight other children (6). The Bertrams and Mrs. Norris do appear snobbish and self-congratulatory (we are never meant to assume that they are morally superior to the Prices), but they seem more capable of raising healthy children. The vigilant patriarch, Sir Thomas, looks out for the harm Fanny's residence might cause his own family, warning Mrs. Norris that "[s]hould [Fanny's] disposition be really bad, . . . we must not, for our own children's sake, continue her in the family" (10). This concern about her "disposition" refers initially to Fanny's presumed "bad" manners (a result of her lower class) and the potential problems a bad disposition may cause for the household. It assumes, as well, that things at Mansfield Park are fine as they are.

Disposition is tricky, though, because it evokes both "a frame of mind" and a "state of bodily health" (*Oxford English Dictionary*). The term aligns the moral and the medical, a pairing that underwrites the preventionist interest in domestic management. When Sir Thomas uses *disposition* to describe what Fanny could be (but probably is not) like, he invokes the specter of prevention, imagining what might need to be avoided at a future date. He explains to Mrs. Norris that they are likely to encounter "gross ignorance, some meanness of opinion, and very distressing vulgarity of manner." Such conduct, he determines, is neither "incurable" nor "dangerous" to those around her, and although he refers here to "curing" her habits, he does so in a preemptive manner, thinking of keeping his children disease-free rather than of helping Fanny to improve (10). His language shifts our focus from the social to the physical, from her behavior to her body, and Mrs. Price's letter reaffirms this dual meaning.[21] She offers "assur[ance] of her daughter's being a very well-disposed, good-humoured girl" but then confirms the alternative meaning of *disposition* when she shares her hope that her daughter's health will improve as a result of her contact with Mansfield Park's salubrious "air" (11). The novel's interest in Fanny's improvement, however, never fully materializes, as key episodes that appear to feature her as the heroine of a cure plot turn, instead, on her preventionist perspective.

In fact, we are encouraged from very early on to see Fanny as a struggling preventionist. When the "old grey poney[*sic*]" she has been used to riding dies, the narrator tells us that Fanny "was in danger of feeling the loss in her health as well as her affections" (31). Nobody thinks to replace her pony until Edmund, the only one to attend to Fanny's physical well-being, notices the loss's "ill effects" (32) and trades his road horse for a suitable mare. The lack of both a horse and the family's interest in getting Fanny a horse contributes to her potential decline. Medically speaking, horseback riding, or some comparable activity, was often prescribed as therapeutic during this period. For example, Buchan observes that "exercise is not less necessary than food for the preservation of health" and that "[i]t seems to be a catholic law throughout the whole animal creation, that no creature, without exercise, should enjoy health, or be able to find subsistence."[22] Not surprisingly, riding makes Fanny feel better, and without it she is in danger of getting sick again. But this episode, we know, is not about proclaiming the benefits of a particular medical regimen. Rather, it demonstrates Fanny's desire for Edmund, a desire that Austen presents as prevention. When Edmund lends Mary Crawford the mare, we see instantly what must be avoided—and it is not Fanny's ill health. The horse shifts our attention from Fanny's need for improvement to Edmund's more pressing need for intervention.

The static and "delicate" Fanny needs somehow to hinder the seemingly healthier "active and fearless" Mary Crawford from winning her cousin's affections, but this task is not easy. As Fanny watches from a distance, waiting for Edmund and Mary to return with the horse, she "[feels] a pang" at the thought that Edmund should forget her. The narrator never goes so far as to describe Fanny as jealous, an emotion that would place her firmly in a therapeutic plot. But we do learn that Edmund and Mary's "merriment ascended even to [Fanny]," and "[i]t was a sound which did not make *her* cheerful" (57). When Edmund asks Fanny for permission to lend Mary the horse, he assures Fanny that her health has priority over Mary's pleasure. "It would be very wrong," he explains, for Mary to "interfere" with Fanny's regimen: "*She* rides only for pleasure, *you* for health" (59). At this point, the novel moves rather comfortably between the medical and the metaphorical, as Fanny's literal health offers Edmund a way to talk about Mary's (and presumably his own) desire. Fanny must acquiesce—it is, after all, Edmund's horse. But more to the point, she must give up the horse because she does not want Edmund to think of her as continually incapacitated and thus unfit to participate in a love plot of her own. When his only excuse for Fanny's riding is her health, she reminds him that she is "strong enough now to walk very well" (59). For Edmund, the horse represents a narrative of Fanny's perpetual cure. For Fanny, the horse incites a narrative of Edmund's prevented affections. In both cases, prevention prevails, but it is not until the Sotherton episode that we see prevention at work and Fanny as its most active agent.

Significantly, Austen does not frame the Sotherton excursion and Fanny's warning at the ha-ha as a moment of crisis in need of cure; she frames it in terms of advancing prevention and of Fanny's highly developed foresight. Fanny is static, sitting on her bench in the wilderness because she has become too fatigued to walk. Fanny can only, therefore, watch Edmund and Mary walk off to "determine the dimension of the wood" (81) and Maria and Henry slip dangerously over the ha-ha. We experience, through Fanny, the desire of anticipation, imagining what might be, as her condition forces her to remain on the bench while both of these couples wander unchaperoned among the shrubs. Initially, Fanny attempts to stop Edmund and Mary from leaving her, but she gets rebuffed: "Edmund urged her [to] remai[n] where she was with an earnestness which she could not resist." The narrator tells us that "she was left on the bench to think with pleasure of her cousin's care, but with great regret that she was not stronger" (81). At this moment, Edmund does not want her and neither do we, because she hinders us from following the more illicit, narratable couples, the ones who will get into trouble, create conflict, and need curing. But this is precisely how prevention functions as narrative, for all Fanny can do at this point, and all Austen really wants her to do, is watch so that, as readers, we are left to anticipate rather than to witness what ought not happen.

Austen expands Fanny's preventionist reach by redirecting Fanny's efforts away from Edmund and Mary and toward the more dangerous coupling of Maria Bertram and Henry Crawford. Rather than actively prevent anything from happening (for, as I have noted, she will fail), Fanny allows us to imagine what, in the words of Marianne Dashwood, "ought to have been." Her warnings reflect three very good reasons for Maria to stop her current behavior: "'You will hurt yourself Miss Bertram,' she cried, 'You will certainly hurt yourself against those spikes—you will tear your gown—you will be in danger of slipping into the Ha-Ha'" (84). The first and last arguments refer to preventing bodily injury. All three hint at the real reason for Fanny's concern—Maria's virtue is at risk. Perhaps Fanny should have taken a cue from Dr. Beddoes and warned Maria that she will most certainly become a wretch if she travels down this path—but would Maria have listened? That seems unlikely. Certainly one thing is clear: Fanny cannot stop what she is sure will (and what, in fact, does) lead only to mischief and heartache.

Maria's unfortunate end is less a failure of prevention than a failure of cure—the cure that sets out to turn Henry Crawford from a rake into a good husband. Prevention is never given a chance. Readers have been reluctant to recognize this point and to subscribe to a preventionist ethos, because, like most of the characters in *Mansfield Park*, readers actually prefer disaster, always needing the fix of a "cure" to keep them interested. Busily reading for a fall ("you will slip"), they want bad behavior to proceed and then be fixed. But readers, too, are insufficiently cautious—they eagerly read ahead when they should be carefully reading backward. And for this reason, Austen aligns her plan of prevention with a plot of temporal displacement, one that "cautions" its readers. We see this arrangement in the great (failed) cure of the novel: Sir Thomas's attempt to "cure" Fanny by sending her home to Portsmouth. This episode sends us backward into the novel, teaching us why Fanny is the one who will triumph in the end. Our removal to Portsmouth in the final volume shows us, in fact, what has already been prevented.

It is no accident that Sir Thomas is the great believer in cure—after all, he is the novel's worst preventionist, as we know from watching his children misbehave, fall, and fall ill. The second half of *Mansfield Park* is Sir Thomas's attempt to cure his physically healthy but morally diseased family. To do so, he sends Fanny home—but he also sends readers into the past, where Austen not only exhibits Fanny's spiritual fortitude but also teaches readers how to read preventatively. Sir Thomas returns Fanny to Portsmouth and to her "mismanaged family" to teach her a lesson, introducing us to characters we have met only through narration and epistolarity. As with her entrance into Mansfield, Fanny's homecoming is imagined as a "medicinal project" (305). Sir Thomas hopes that sending her away from her upper-middle-class environs will "cure" her "diseased" understanding and make her appreciate Henry Crawford's marriage proposal. And in part, he is right. What she finds when she arrives at Portsmouth is a house full of unruly children, ill-trained servants, and greasy dishes. As the narrator explains, "It was an abode of noise, disorder, and impropriety" (322). More than three hundred pages after our initial introduction to the Price family, we feel for the first time the burden that nine pregnancies and a "husband disabled for active service" (6) must be. We meet a drunken father who fails to notice his daughter, and a mother who is too busy with her eight other children to be more than merely "not unkind" (323). The narrator shifts allegiances here, for at the end of the opening chapter of volume 1, we are encouraged to sympathize with the "[p]oor woman" who just wants her children to be well. Fanny's chief antagonist, Mrs. Norris, now appears positively maternal when compared to Mrs. Price.

Prevention narratives are designed for precisely the type of parents Fanny has endured, and Mr. Price is as much of a cautionary tale as is his wife. Not only does he show little interest in his daughter's well-being and absolutely no interest in Mansfield but also he has no authority in his home. Fanny's first point of comparison with Sir Thomas is the fact that all her father can talk about is William going away: "[I]n her uncle's house there would have been a consideration of times and seasons, a regulation of subject, a propriety, an attention toward every body which there was not here" (317). But more than lacking the ability or desire to properly direct conversation, Mr. Price has none of the patriarchal control that Sir Bertram seems to enjoy. His empty threats are, as Fanny notices, "palpably disregarded" by the noisy young boys, who only quiet down after they appear to have worn themselves out. In his earlier manual, *A Guide for Self Preservation, and Parental Affection* (1793), Beddoes asserts, "To keep the children strong, and in good plight to stand such complaints [measles, sore throat, fever, or any other violent disorder], there is but one way. The father must be sober and industrious; and the mother learn to manage well."[23] The Prices fail on all accounts.

The lackluster greeting mimics the narrative logic of prevention by showing us what would have been Fanny's whole life—and so it could still be, if Sir Thomas has his way. But Fanny is initially disconnected from Portsmouth. She looked forward with pleasure to her homecoming, imagining a more affectionate relationship with her mother than she had experienced in the past, despite William's warning that "we seem to want some of your nice ways and orderliness" (308). Her return to Portsmouth turns out to be less a homecoming than a first-time visit. The narrator describes the route William and Fanny take to get to the house with none of the nostalgic reminiscences one might expect from someone of Fanny's sensibility. After all, she is the one who turns to Cowper when she imagines the "avenue" at Sotherton (a place she has never seen) being "cut down" (48). We hear no such lamentations or recollections of the past from Fanny upon her first seeing Portsmouth after being away for nine years. The narrator tells us that Fanny and William "were rattled into a narrow street . . . and drawn up before the door of a small house now inhabited by Mr. Price" (312). This description suggests that Fanny, like the reader, is seeing the house for the first time. It is not "their" small house or "the" house but rather "a" house. The "now" adds to the ambiguity, implying at first that Mr. Price is at that present moment in the house but also suggesting that Mr. Price and the Price family formerly inhabited another house—the house Fanny grew up in—and "now" inhabit this one. Upon entering the house, Fanny confuses the parlor for "a passage-room" (because it is so small), and later Mrs. Price complains about the inconvenience of not having a "butcher in the street," noting that "[w]e were better off in our last house" (313, 314). This "we" does not appear to include Fanny. Mrs. Price's complaint serves as a general comment to anyone who will listen about her dissatisfaction but also suggests quite simply that Fanny does not know this particular street—this is not her home.

Recounting Fanny's Portsmouth life through estrangement and structural disorder allows Austen to invoke a preventionist—or what I refer to elsewhere as a "hygienic"—mode of reading and thinking. We need to see Portsmouth as a new place in order for this return to feel more like an originary moment, a moment that has "come before" earlier episodes, before Mary rode her pony and before Maria jumped the ha-ha. This return does not stand in completely for Fanny's past. Certainly, a lot has happened since she last lived at Portsmouth: the babies have grown into adolescents, two more have been born, and William is no longer her companion. However, whether the place to which Fanny returns is her former home or whether it is more chaotic than it once was is not at issue. The basic condition—the domestic mismanagement—we witness during Fanny's return replicates that which made Fanny's initial "change of air" so desirable. And once again, Portsmouth makes Fanny sick, as we are told that "she had lost ground as to health since her being in Portsmouth" (339). Not only does Fanny reject Portsmouth, but Portsmouth rejects Fanny. The house virtually squeezes her out, almost suffocating her with "the smallness of the rooms" and "the narrowness of the passage and staircase" (321). Inactivity and lack of air accelerate her decline, such that when Henry Crawford comes to visit, he feels compelled to explain to Susan that Fanny "requires constant air and exercise" and that "she ought never to be long banished from the free air, and liberty of the country" (340). Because this scene takes place after Fanny has been living at Mansfield, we initially read Fanny's decline as a psychosomatic response to her separation from Edmund and as evidence of her altered disposition. But Henry's reference to "free air" recalls Mrs. Price's initial hope that Fanny will be "materially better for change of air," thus collapsing, if only momentarily, narrative time and allowing us to read the Fanny of volume 3 as the Fanny from volume 1. This situation is the very one that paradoxically fortified her against Mansfield and helped to establish Fanny as an agent of prevention.

Austen offers a particularly telling story of mismanagement and prevention in this final volume, one that, like the Elizas in *Sense and Sensibility*, haunts (has haunted all along) the narrative. Shortly after Fanny came to Mansfield Park, her favorite sister died. Austen withholds the news of Mary Price's death until we are in Portsmouth and see the conditions under which the sister lived. We never get to witness Fanny's response, learning only during her return to Portsmouth that when she found out, she "had for a short time been quite afflicted" (320). We can read Fanny's sorrow back into the narrative, speculating that it occurred somewhere between Mrs. Norris's haranguing, Maria and Julia's teasing, and Edmund's care. At the same time, Mrs. Price's wish that her children might be "materially better" becomes more firmly grounded in bodily health. Fanny's move to Mansfield (the "change of air") may have prevented her own death, but more than that—more than being the silent recipient of preventive care—Fanny's change of space (the movement from Mansfield Park to Portsmouth) registers as a temporal shift. The move allows Austen to compress time and revise our imperfect knowledge about Fanny's early life. Austen's placement of the Portsmouth episode at the end trains us to see both what has come before and what could be. We can apply this thinking to Fanny's attachment to Edmund and to her observations of his relationship with Mary Crawford.

After walking in the Sotherton woods, Edmund and Mary become the main characters in Fanny's prevention tale. Edmund is headed down a slippery path that nobody has taught him to traverse, for he has been mesmerized by Mary's manipulative ways—enough to make him partake in the acting "scheme" he initially condemned (128). But Fanny has been watching and, in a sense, narrating for us the danger that awaits him were he to marry a woman who has no desire to be a clergyman's wife. Through her, we anticipate Edmund looking back at this moment with regret. Of course, we also know that it will not culminate in this way. When Edmund finally realizes that the woman he courted was not "Miss Crawford" but only "the creature of [his] own imagination" (378), we sense some of what has been averted. This change, however, reflects minimal growth. His "impulse . . . to resist" Mary's "saucy playful smile" is slightly contaminated by his admission that he "sometimes—for a moment—regretted that [he] did not go back" to Mary (379). For even though he has witnessed her deception, he still fantasizes about "how excellent she would have been, had she fallen into good hands earlier" (379). Here, Edmund puts a preventionist ethic to potentially dangerous use, imagining Mary as what she might have been and turning her into the woman he would have married. Mary is a cautionary wretch, and Fanny puts an end to Edmund's revisionist fantasy by "adding to his knowledge of [Mary's] real character." She explains to him that Tom's ill health and thus the potential for Edmund (as the younger son) to be heir appealed to Mary. Austen reveals Edmund's response to this "hint" through the narrator's ambiguous observation that "[t]his was not an agreeable intimation. Nature resisted it for a while." But only for a while. Eventually, outside of the narrative, he grows out of his fantasy—"his vanity was not of a strength to fight long against reason"—and he sees as he ought and chooses Fanny (379).

With Edmund on the proper path and Fanny poised to be his companion, two important questions remain: What, exactly, has been prevented in *Mansfield Park?* And more pressingly, how do we achieve closure through prevention? Medically speaking, the one serious illness in the novel is not prevented and, in fact, becomes an important plot point. Tom Bertram's condition brings Fanny back from Portsmouth so that she can comfort the Bertrams and expose Mary Crawford.[24] But even as Tom's story reflects a discourse of cure, it does so within a larger framework of prevention; he, like Maria and Julia Bertram and Mary Price, becomes a cautionary tale about the dangers of debauchery and of bad parenting. Tom's illness and recovery enable him to "bec[o]me what he ought to be, useful to his father, steady and quiet, and not merely living for himself" (381); Maria must be sacrificed to the story of prevention, while her sister, though initially wretched, gets a reprieve. The narrator explains that Sir Thomas finally becomes "conscious of errors in his own conduct as a parent" and is "the longest to suffer." Only in hindsight—because he lacked the foresight—does he realize what he "ought not to have" done (380). He comforts himself, however, with the notion that his own daughters' "real dispositions [were] unknown to him" (381). His strictness was no match for Mrs. Norris's schemes, yet he refuses to take full blame for their "real disposition," reasoning that "something must have been wanting *within*" (382). While Sir Thomas refers to their moral failing, his language (in light of the eldest son's sickness) is partly medical, reminding us of his early concerns about Fanny's disposition. Having been trained by Austen as preventionist readers, we know, however, that had Sir Thomas looked beneath the healthy surface and the pleasing manners of his children, he might have seen the "disease" growing within, for the moral and the medical, as Beddoes makes clear, are of a piece.

The novel does not spend much time worrying over these obvious examples of what has and has not been prevented, because it is rather more interested in Edmund's case. Has he been prevented from marrying the wrong woman or merely "cure[d]" of what the narrator calls "unconquerable passion" (387)? After all, the Crawfords have been described as needing "cure," and, moreover, because they do not "wan[t] to be cured" (40), Mary's status as potentially infectious remains open. We might even give Mary credit for inoculating Edmund—his limited contact with the morally tainted Mary helps to fortify Edmund against future "disease" and keep him healthy for Fanny. Austen's language in the pivotal exchange between Edmund and Fanny—that his "nature" resisted the truth and that he only recognized Fanny's worth when it was "natural" for him to do so—suggests that Edmund was never really "sick," that Fanny's preventive project (her presence) worked: it preserved Edmund's naturally healthy disposition and has protected him from future wretchedness.

Indeed, Edmund's epiphany implies that Fanny has been his guide and protector all the while he imagined himself to be hers. The narrator explains, "With such a regard for her, indeed, as his had long been, a regard founded on the most endearing claims of innocence and helplessness, and completed by every recommendation of growing worth, what could be more natural than the change? Loving, guiding, protecting her, as he had been doing ever since her being ten years old, her mind so great a degree formed by his care, and her comfort depending on his kindness, an object to him of such close and peculiar interest, dearer by all his own importance with her than any one else at Mansfield" (387). Edmund's claim to have been "loving, guiding, [and] protecting" Fanny since she was ten does not account for the unintentional neglect she suffered at his hands, giving her horse to Mary or leaving her on the bench at Sotherton. His version of the story is slightly inaccurate. We know, too, that without Fanny's "hint," his nature could not have detected Mary's "real character"; it would have only fantasized about her excellence and his loss. Austen means for us to speculate about what could have been, as the narrator states explicitly that "had [Henry] done as he intended, and as he knew he ought, . . . he might have been deciding his own happy destiny" (385). Mary takes a slightly different view, blaming Fanny for Henry's bad behavior. She tells Edmund that Fanny "would have fixed" Henry, and "[h]ad she accepted him as she ought, they might now have been on the point of marriage" and Henry would not have eloped with Maria Bertram, now Maria Rushworth (376). But however much Mary or the reader may wish for this alternative ending, the narrative has never been interested in curing Henry Crawford because it was never interested in the Fanny-Henry plot—it was never interested in cure. Nor has it been interested in protecting the other Bertram children, whose stories, as Beddoes might say, only "pretend to teach people how to restore [health]."[25] Rather, the narrative has always been concerned with advancing Fanny's desire for Edmund and the preventionist stance that such desire represents.

To answer the question of how we achieve closure through prevention, I return to the physicians. Buchan has difficulty addressing prevention's narrative constraints about an end. And for all his emphasis on prophylaxis, he concludes by offering a list of cures, beginning with balsams and ending with wines. Beddoes, in contrast, concludes his final installment by explaining that there is no conclusion. He maintains, "There yet remain many subjects in preventive medicine," and he goes on to express what we know or hope to be true of our favorite writers—namely, that they will have more to offer. "I find myself," he says, "far from spent with the toil, and I can say with as good a heart as many who have lain by, all the time, in the shade—'To-morrow to fresh woods and pastures new.'"[26] We must always be vigilant about maintaining health.

The novelist provides the rest of the answer. The curt, and what one critic calls "controversial,"[27] ending of *Mansfield Park* disrupts the kind of tidy restoration generally offered by cure. The narrator blunts the certainty of closure by rushing to assure us that "[m]y Fanny indeed at this very time, I have the satisfaction of knowing, must have been happy in spite of every thing. She must have been a happy creature in spite of all that she felt or thought she felt, for the distress of those around her. She has sources of delight that must force their way" (380). The narrator is, perhaps, too emphatic about Fanny's happiness. The repetition of "must" is as much an assertion of what will occur as it is a question about what should happen—Fanny *must* be happy after all that she has endured, mustn't she?

Of course she must. But not immediately. The narrator "purposely abstain[s]" from telling us when Fanny became happy, instead "intreat[ing] every body to believe that exactly at the time when it was quite natural that it should be so, and not a week earlier, Edmund did cease to care about Mary Crawford, and became as anxious to marry Fanny, as Fanny herself could desire" (387). What some see as an uncharacteristically rushed and overly personal conclusion, Tony Tanner sees as a transfer of the "obligation of the author to the discretion (or fantasy) of the reader"; the absence of specificity becomes an invitation to "write *this* part of the novel."[28] Though Tanner refers here to Austen's refusal to depict Edmund and Fanny in conjugal bliss or something quite like it—"they are after all cousins"[29]—I see this gesture toward the development of the reader's imaginative capacity as coincident with the project of prevention.

Cure and restoration are important to narrative, but as *Sense and Sensibility* and *Mansfield Park* show us, the stories that come before and beyond cure, the ones that carry us outside of a recovery model, are equally valuable, though perhaps not quite as exciting. Prevention, as I have been suggesting, is a way of reading; it is a lesson in patience more than it is a lesson in being a patient. Elinor Dashwood is arguably Austen's first preventionist heroine, while Fanny Price, the sickly central heroine who is not trying to get well, is perhaps her most complex. Even her final complete novel, *Persuasion,* suggests that prevention more than cure guides our reading. The invalid Mrs. Smith registers the kind of anticipatory regret that prevention seeks to instill. But in *Persuasion,* we also get a turn away from prevention, for Anne Elliot, who lost her bloom before the novel begins and regains it before our very eyes, seems to argue against preventionist thinking, not because it lacks the narrative force of cure but because it is too much like it. Having followed Lady Russell's advice and turned down Wentworth's proposal eight years before the novel begins, Anne, though longing to regain her lost love, does not blame herself for following this advice. She does, however, feel that "were any young person, in similar circumstances, to apply to her for counsel, they would never receive any of such certain immediate wretchedness, such uncertain future good" (20). In Anne's situation, prevention, instead of mitigating wretchedness, becomes the only way to ensure it.

Telling the story of prevention is not easy. In real life, we are left to recognize the signs and structure of preventive thinking and to do our best to avoid what we are sure *might* cause us harm. In fiction, we get a bit more insight, a bit more certainty, as the narrator can tell us (if she so chooses) what might have been. But even in fiction, prevention is still a shadow, an imagined story of averted future regret that hovers over all the stories we tell.

Chapter Two

Health, Identity, and Narrative Authority in *Jane Eyre*

> Q. 10. The blessings of health then must be very great?
>
> A. They are indeed. Health is the most precious good, and the most certain means of enjoying all other blessings and pleasures of life.
>
> Q. 11. What says the son of Sirach of health?
>
> A. . . . "Better is the poor being sound and strong of constitution, than a rich man that is afflicted in his body. Health and good estate of body are above all gold, and a strong body above infinite wealth. There are no riches above a sound body, and no joy above the joy of the heart."
>
> —Bernhard Christoph Faust, M.D.,
> *The Catechism of Health* (1794)

> "And what is hell? Can you tell me that?"
> "A pit full of fire."
> "And should you like to fall into that pit, and to be burning for ever?"
> "No, sir."
> "What must you do to avoid it?"
> I deliberated a moment: my answer, when it did come, was objectionable: "I must keep in good health, and not die."
> "How can you keep in good health? Children younger than you die daily."
>
> —Charlotte Brontë, *Jane Eyre* (1847)

Young Jane Eyre's assertion that she must "keep in good health" has more in common with Faust's "Catechism of Health" than it does with Reverend Brocklehurst's interrogation about hell.[1] The reverend's doctrine of mortification, which is best exemplified by his mismanagement of Lowood, dismisses health as untenable and declares "worldly happiness" to be dangerous. Jane's answer, therefore, is grossly uninformed, a symptom of her wickedness, stupidity, and obstinacy. The reader, of course does not see it quite this way, instead interpreting Jane's reply as simply naïve or too literal, an honest response to a rigged question. But as Jane tells her story, and as her attempts to heed her own advice become intertwined with its telling, her rejoinder proves to be more savvy than we might first have appreciated; certainly it is more attuned to the exigencies of the world than is Brocklehurst's subsequent parable of the sickly, psalm-loving child. The gap between Brocklehurst's and Jane's perspectives—health is nothing versus health is everything—signals more than a theological divide between a hypocritical clergyman and a willful young girl.[2] It draws attention to a crucial epistemological concern circulating throughout the nineteenth century that underwrites the physician's authority to offer advice about and define health and the novelist's capacity to intervene in this endeavor. The Reverend Brocklehurst may not care about health, but Jane certainly does—and so should we. Her story, I am suggesting, functions as an extended answer to this complex question: How can you keep in good health?

The question of whether keeping in good health is possible looms large in the cultural imagination, and the answer offered by medical advisers of the period was a qualified yes. One can keep well, but it takes work. Eating the right foods, breathing fresh air, getting proper rest, and moderate exercise go a long way toward preserving health, but not everyone has the means or opportunity to take such care. And even if they did, deadly epidemics and inherited disease have a way of interfering with the best-laid plans. The Brontës' own tragic family history attests to this reality: Charlotte's mother and two of her sisters died when she was a child; the rest of her siblings died within a year and a half after the publication of *Jane Eyre.*[3] Her father, the Reverend Patrick Brontë, took copious notes on the vicissitudes of his and his children's health. He worked diligently to keep them well and to find cures when they were not. As Sally Shuttleworth points out in her pioneering study *Charlotte Brontë and Victorian Psychology,* Reverend Brontë's "fascination with medical science, and the inter-relations between the mind and the body, went far beyond the bounds of professional duty, . . . leading him to impose a rigorous regime on his entire family. Every symptom, whether of mental or physical ill-health, was closely scrutinized, and checked against the near-infallible words of his secular Bible, Graham's *Domestic Medicine.*"[4]

Reverend Brontë's "bible," like Faust's catechism, promises to educate readers about the importance of health. In Faust's case, the lesson takes the form of a repetitive performance in the hope that it will become a habit. Students must recite the catechism for "an hour, twice a week," so that "the minds of the children [become] *impressed* with the true spirit of its doctrine":[5] health is a blessing, and preserving it is one's duty. The problem for those who write about health is not only that medical knowledge about the body is uncertain and faulty but also that readers must be conditioned to take an interest in their health; they must work to cultivate a sense of health in order to keep it. John Milner Fothergill begins his *Maintenance of Health* (1874) by acknowledging this problem. He explains, "What is attempted here is to give such information about 'the casket of the soul' as will enable the lay reader to have some idea of his own frame and its physiology, and by describing what health is, and how variations from it are brought about, to give him some general impressions as to what to do in order to be well and to keep well."[6] The directive—know health and keep well—reverberates throughout *Jane Eyre* and throughout Victorian culture, becoming a defining feature of the stories Victorians told to and about themselves.

Narrative theorists have noted the importance of stories to identity formation. And as *Jane Eyre* demonstrates so well, these stories owe something to our sense of physical wellness.[7] Our definition of health, in other words, is a definition of self and thus plays a significant role in the form and content of the tales we tell. Jane defines herself as rebellious and romantic. Hers, therefore, is a story about social inequality and about love; it is both a "radical feminist assertion of female autonomy"[8] and a courtship narrative par excellence.[9] Brontë draws these two narrative strands (rebellion and romance) together with Jane's simple assertion that she must "keep in good health," a refrain that acts as her finest weapon against injustice and a dictum around which her marriage plot unfolds.

As a novel that aligns narrative authority with the capacity to maintain good health, *Jane Eyre* both exemplifies and resolves some of the challenges that medical writers face when warning readers to value health's presence rather than to regret its absence or mourn its loss. For while the therapeutic narrative is, indeed, part of the organizing structure of the novel, it is not, I would argue, the primary dynamic at work in Jane's story. Jane is not looking for literal or figurative cures. Even as the novel's plot (orphan girl turned governess becomes an heiress and finds happiness in marriage) encourages our desire to read for such closure, Brontë repeatedly disrupts this traditional narrative structure in favor of one less concerned with its end.[10] As much as it builds toward "Reader, I married him," *Jane Eyre* simultaneously trains readers to be suspicious of such narrative "cures" and to interpret Jane's sustained—or mostly sustained—health as a model of reading that demands patience and delays, or even denies, the gratification that comes from cure.

The battle between these two modes (therapeutic and hygienic) modes of reading emerges early in the novel, before young Jane has developed what Thomas Beddoes refers to as "health sense." When confronted by Brocklehurst's accusation—"How can you keep in good health?"—Jane can only sigh and get into more trouble.

Brocklehurst and Mrs. Reed mark Jane as metaphorically diseased and in need of cure. The reverend knows she is bound for hell, because Mrs. Reed has offered evidence that she is wicked and because Jane has revealed, through her preferred Bible verses ("Psalms are not interesting"), that she "must have a wicked heart" (40). Jane cannot argue points of spirituality or religion with Brocklehurst, but she can assert what will hold her and her plot in good stead: she is remarkably healthy. At Lowood, she identifies with the minority that survives typhus; at Thornfield, Edward Rochester deems her "an instrument of [his] cure" (99); at Moor House, St. John Rivers does not let her die, whereas in India he would have (496); and at the "insalubrious site" of Ferndean Manor, she finds "perfect concord" (519).

Given the historical realities of the period, this record of health is no small feat.[11] As Miriam Bailin argues in *The Sickroom in Victorian Fiction*, "One need only look at the grim facts of Charlotte Brontë's life to account for the ubiquity in her novels of states of fever, debility, hypochondria, and morbid decline."[12] Bailin explains that sickness is often "the primary form of self-assertion, convalescence the measure of comfort, and physical dependency the enabling condition of intimacy."[13] But where Bailin reads "somatic disorder" as central to Brontë's novels, particularly *Shirley*, I see, at least in *Jane Eyre*, a desire to sustain somatic order and ordering. Disease is everywhere, but each time Jane's story gets drawn into a therapeutic mode of thinking and reading, she redoubles her effort to cultivate health and to imagine existing outside of a system that has the authority to define her through diagnosis, treatment, and cure. Physical health and the independence and pleasure it produces inform not only what Jane tells about herself but also how she tells it.

From the beginning, Jane's authority depends, in part, on her capacity to frame health—its maintenance and meaning—as resistance not only to disease but also to the narrative structures that fail to accommodate health's complexity and, by extension, her own. When Jane recovers from her red-room fit, Brontë connects Jane's desire to narrate—her compulsion to tell her story—to an impulse for health.[14] Jane overhears Abbot comment that Mrs. Reed will be glad to "get rid of such a tiresome, ill-conditioned child, who always looked as if she were watching everybody, and scheming plots underhand," and thus she learns "for the first time" about her parents' history (31). By juxtaposing Jane's skills as a narrator (her plotting) with her parents' tragic plot, Brontë establishes Jane's desire to preserve health as a concomitant desire for narrative, a desire that begins more simply as a choice between death and survival.

When Jane chooses not to starve herself in protest of her red-room incarceration, she asserts an explicit desire to live and, beyond that, demonstrates a burgeoning awareness of what it means to keep well. Her question to Bessie "Am I ill?" develops the "health sense" that will guide Jane throughout her story. Bessie answers with a hesitant, "You fell sick, I suppose, in the red-room with crying" (24). Her tentative and perhaps skeptical "I suppose," coupled with her fear (which Jane overhears) that Jane "might die" as a result of her "strange" fit, teach Jane that she must begin to answer such questions for herself. Mr. Lloyd, the apothecary who attends Jane after her "fit," gives Jane the opportunity to do just that when he asks her, "What made you ill yesterday?" Bessie tries to answer for Jane, explaining that she fell, but Jane corrects Bessie in two ways: first, she states that she did not fall, she was knocked down; then she rejects the assumption that she cannot endure physical trauma, explaining, "[T]hat did not make me ill," it was being "shut up in a room where there is a ghost." The doctor's strategy for "curing" Jane is simply to point out that she is too old for such "nonsense": "What, you are a baby after all?" he asks playfully. Although Jane holds to her concerns about the ghost, this encounter with the doctor is her "first opportunity of relieving her grief," which she attempts to do as truthfully as she can. She tells of her mistreatment, and adopting the doctor's own language of maturation, she laments that she "can never get away from Gateshead till [she is] a woman" (29). The journey from infancy to womanhood, like the journey from Gateshead to Ferndean, is a treacherous one. And above all, it requires one to stay healthy. To do that, however, either one must be highly attentive to one's body and environment or one must turn, as I do briefly, to the advice of the professionals who presumably know better.

MEDICAL ADVICE AND THE MEANING OF HEALTH

Jane's response to Reverend Brocklehurst that she must "keep in good health" seemed obvious enough to Jane, but what did "good health" mean to the Victorians reading *Jane Eyre* and what were the rhetorical strategies that medical writers used in their attempts to teach readers, like Jane, what health is? The simple answer, the one with which nineteenth-century readers might have most identified, is that health is, as Samuel Johnson's *Dictionary of the English Language* (1755) puts it, "[f]reedom from bodily pain or sickness."[15] Explaining what health is *not,* however, does not explain what it is. Health, in Johnson's formulation, is an absence. Disease, by contrast, is the presence of something: Johnson defines disease as "distemper, malady, sickness, morbid state."[16] Admittedly, this somewhat tautological definition offers its own rhetorical challenges, but most medical manuals and specialized treatises provide detailed descriptions, sometimes contradictory, of various diseases (such as cholera, smallpox, tuberculosis, and fevers of all sorts).[17] We can learn about their causes, etiologies, and cures and presumably know what they are, even if that knowledge is, as often history bears out, wrong. Health, it would seem, is the absence of the symptoms of disease or awareness of its presence in the body.

While defining health as not-disease provides a framework within which we might begin to know health, it does not tell a complete or compelling story. Contemporary medical writers note that it seems logical to define health as the "absence of disease or illness," but it is more productive to see health as "refer[ring] to something more."[18] Eighteenth- and nineteenth-century writers were similarly aware of the limitations of such a rigid binary. Citing medical writer John Quincy, Samuel Johnson implies in the extended definition (which was cut from the abridged version) that this "something more" involves "the faculty of performing all actions proper to a human body, in the most perfect manner." Following humoral theories of medicine—that the body is in a state of health when all vital fluids (humors) are balanced[19]—Quincy depicts health as the presence of "proper" action. Of course, determining what counts as "proper" or normal, as Michel Foucault and others have demonstrated, becomes a way to pathologize and demonize socially or politically objectionable activities, experiences, and conditions. Pamela Gilbert has recently demonstrated, for example, that for nineteenth-century sanitary reformers "[h]ealth was defined as a set of hygienic practices that created a bodily habitus appropriate to the development of middle-class tastes."[20]

But within these attempts to discipline readers to read properly for health and to become good (morally and literally clean) middle-class citizens, writers' definitions reveal as well the possibilities for resisting any single interpretation. The discourse surrounding health oscillates between empowerment and oppression, between commonsense tips for keeping well and directives for preserving the status quo or promoting new social norms. As Johnson's friend the physician Robert James notes in his popular three-volume *A Medicinal Dictionary* (1743) (to which Johnson contributed entries), health "is very rare, and even perhaps never to be met with." We can only "suppose or imagine such a Model for regulating our Judgments, with respect to less perfect constitutions."[21] Envisioning what could or should be becomes just as important to the definition of health as the experience itself. In fact, imagining health and behaving in ways that preserve that imagined state might be all one can do. Even Fothergill can only promise to instruct his reader in the "maintenance . . . not of ideal health, but the best possible health to the individual."[22] As William Strange puts it in his *Seven Sources of Health* (1864), "Health is a mere abstraction, made up of a variety of ideal images which present themselves in a different guise to the mind of almost every individual."[23]

J. H. Walsh's definition makes a similar point about the imaginative demands health makes on readers when he articulates health's variability in his *Manual of Domestic Medicine and Surgery* (1858):

> Sect 1.—Definition of Health
> 1. In the present artificial state of society, the health, both of individuals and [of] communities, is always comparative, none of us being quite free from the ill effects upon our constitutions, of excess in the indulgence of our appetites, or the influence of bad air, defective drainage or mental excitement upon our nervous systems. Just as it is almost impossible to find a perfectly sound horse in this country, because we all have a "screw loose" somewhere, so a human being with a "sound mind in a sound body" is equally a "rara avis."

He goes on to qualify this claim:

> But in common language, we are accustomed to use the term "good health" as meaning that state of the system which is the average condition of those who are free from absolute disease. The different degrees of health ascend from "good" to "strong" and "perfect," which is the highest term used; while below the average the adjectives "pretty fair," "delicate," "feeble," "bad," and "very bad" mark the descending scale—the last term being of course only applicable to those who are the subjects of disease.[24]

Although Walsh's understanding of health still relies, like Johnson's, on disease (or, rather, on its absence), health nonetheless holds the default position—there are "different degrees of health." To be in "very bad" health means to be diseased, implying that we begin, rhetorically, in a state of health and move up or down from there, all of us being at least a little below the line of perfection.

This simple taxonomy enlists the reader's imagination, as we must implicitly construct a story about the potential "effects" of certain behaviors and become savvy about where we fall in the spectrum of possibilities. Failure to assess accurately one's place on this spectrum is dangerous. We see this when Jane Eyre depicts her Aunt Reed's faulty diagnosis of her gluttonous, abusive son, John Reed, as suffering from "delicate health."

When Walsh suggests that health is not one condition but a range of conditions, we are both closer to a meaning of health and further away from knowing what "it" is. "There are," Fothergill notes, "types of health as there are the flesh of the fishes and the flesh of the beasts."[25] And by depicting health as relative to the individual, medical writers privilege singularity. For while advice or "laws" about health often attempt to homogenize behaviors and create a single portrait of *the* healthy body, writers such as William Strange stress variety and individuality. In *The Restoration of Health* (1865), Strange offers that although "[h]ealth, like good, will vary by innumerable shades of difference in the case of each individual, and even in the same person at various times" (8), we still tend to understand it as a single, identifiable state. Like other writers, Strange, who places his emphasis on "restoration" rather than maintenance, defines health in opposition to disease but also acknowledges it as a presence that is relative and rare. In a section titled the "Nature of Disease," for example, he explains, "Disease is the negative or opposite of health, as evil is of good," and he goes on to note, "It is the better qualities, let us hope, which are active and positive; the worse, passive and negative" (8). Health holds an active (narratable) position for Strange, but only tentatively so—we have to "hope" that health dominates.

As with other writers, Strange questions the assumption that health is synonymous with "normal."[26] He concedes in *The Restoration of Health* that "[h]ealth may be, and indeed generally is[,] defined as the *normal* (proper) performance of all functions of the body, that body being organized in a normal manner as regards the type of the race; in other words, the proper action of a good constitution" (8), but he goes on to challenge the usefulness of such a conception: "[W]hen are all the functions duly and perfectly performed? When can we lay our finger upon a period of our lives and say, Now everything is going on within exactly as it should do; now I am in as perfect health as my organization is capable of? Again, who shall say what is a normally constituted frame? Who shall carry off the palm of physical perfection, and make the nearest approach to the Apollo Belvidere? Who shall decide upon the standard of physical beauty or of perfection in the constitutional power?" (9). This series of rhetorical questions turns at last to a metaphor of health as beauty and registers the difficulty of pinpointing what exactly it means to be healthy. Strange implies that health is, essentially, in the eye of the beholder. Instead of being impossible to achieve, health may be achieved by everyone in his or her own way.

By depicting health as particular to the individual but also potentially unattainable, these health "experts" invite their readers to become attentive to the uniqueness and the particularity of their conditions and to tell their own stories—even as the professionals promise to define that uniqueness and tell those stories for them. As individuality and scarcity become integral to one's knowledge of health, one's sense of "what *it* is" expands, becoming more, rather than less, accommodating of difference and deviation. Health is a lived experience (we can feel when we are well), but it is also an ideal state to which we can only aspire (we all have a "screw loose somewhere"). It is relative, various, and just within reach; it is also absolute, specific, and "perhaps never to be met with." Health is both the absence of disease and the presence of proper activity; it is a fiction that requires imaginative, attentive, and patient readers and expert narrators. Jane Eyre is exemplary in both regards: she is a reader and writer of health, as her technique of self-definition—of somatic ordering—typifies the rhetorical strategies and challenges medical writers face when they attempt to define what health is and to teach readers how to maintain it. Jane's "autobiography" reflects an increasingly sophisticated awareness of and interest in her health, as she moves from the limitations imposed by the binaristic thinking we see in Johnson's dictionary toward a more capacious model of self-definition such as the ones developed in later medical writings.

KEEPING WELL IN *Jane Eyre*

Jane's story begins, as Johnson's does, with negation and absence. That is, she learns to define herself as healthy because others depict her as diseased. Brocklehurst is arguably the first to teach Jane the importance of controlling these terms. Not only does he diagnose Jane but also he broadcasts her "illness" to everyone at Lowood. He reads her as a moral toxin and metaphorically diseased, claiming that Jane's "excellent patroness was obliged to separate [Jane] from her own young ones, fearful lest her vicious example should contaminate their purity" and that Jane was sent to Lowood "to be healed, even as the Jews of old sent their diseased to the troubled waters of Bethesda" (79). As such, he first depicts Jane as a public health problem and therefore focuses on prevention. Significantly, Brocklehurst not only invokes prevention falsely but also collapses it into cure: his second claim centers on Jane, rather than the Reeds, and insists on applying the crisis-cure formula to Jane's story—something Jane has engaged in herself.

Prior to Brocklehurst's appearance at the Reeds, Jane claims to be "a discord," "like nobody," out of "harmony," "heterogeneous," "a useless thing," "a noxious thing" (19). Both Jane and Brocklehurst draw on faulty metaphors and an insufficient—because geared toward recovery—narrative structure to encapsulate her experience. Jane is not a disease, nor is she diseased; in fact, in her present environment, being as different from the Reeds as possible is desirable, a sign of literal and metaphorical health. John Reed throws books at little girls, kills pea-chicks, and "gorge[s] himself habitually at the table, which ma[kes] him bilious, and g[ives] him a dim and bleared eye and flabby cheeks" (12). Eliza is "headstrong and selfish," and Georgiana has "a spoiled temper, a very acrid spite, and a captious and insolent carriage" (18). The Reed children, that is, are anything but "pure" examples of good health and minds, strongly suggesting that it is not Jane but they who need to be cured. The irony of these early episodes challenges characters (and critics) who want to diagnose and cure her; these scenes construct—in order to dismantle—the crisis-recovery narrative and the health-illness dichotomy into which others place Jane. The apothecary corrects Brocklehurst's misdiagnosis (that Jane is a liar), and much later in the novel, both Reed sisters prefer Jane's company. Far from being a contaminant, Jane is a balm. But such language, even my own, is too metaphorical. As difficult as it might be, Jane continually resists others' attempts to control her narrative by asserting (not always successfully) medical over metaphorical health.

For Jane, medical health aligns repeatedly with the somatic. And taking control over her narrative means taking control over her body. While medical tracts on health and advice about its maintenance address the important relationship between the mind and the body, particularly in discussing "the passions," Jane's narrative turns on her ability to consciously distinguish between the two, to cordon off mental anguish from physical debility at key moments. In *Charlotte Brontë and Victorian Psychology,* Sally Shuttleworth offers a nuanced reading of Brontë's investment in nineteenth-century psychiatric discourse, arguing that Jane's narrative authority depends largely on her mental status. For Shuttleworth, while questions of "self-control, female body and sexuality, and the insurgence of insanity" hinge on an understanding of the physiological,[27] Jane's narrative effectiveness, she argues, is ultimately governed by her psychological fitness: "Jane's claims to have achieved social success, to have moved out of her initial state of social and psychological marginality, are vindicated by her ability to tell a 'credible' tale and thus win from readers a conviction of her probity and sanity. The measure of her success is the degree to which readers believe we are listening to the workings of 'sane energy,' rather than the ravings of delirium."[28] Jane's desire to maintain "control" of her psyche—to stay sane—appears throughout the novel.

Although Jane's ability to comment retrospectively on her mental anguish certainly lends credibility to her story, I want to address the moments when the psychological imperatives recede and Jane's investment in somatic health dominates. For although mental (which includes moral) and physical health are interdependent and exist less as a binary than along a continuum, Jane and others in her narrative refer repeatedly to the physical and to the material conditions of her body. Jane's strategic separation of physical fitness from mental anguish help to advance her plot when questions about her sanity threaten to dominate and curtail her story. The periodic invocations of bodily health become integral to Jane's storytelling and—to borrow from Shuttleworth—central to Jane's "battle for definitional control."[29] Jane's passionate outbursts and manic internal debates (recall when she puts herself on trial for believing that Rochester would want to marry her) are part of what make the novel so compelling, truthful, and "unVictorian,"[30] but Brontë grounds such episodes in the relatively fit (though petite, pale, and plain) body of her novel's narrator.[31] Jane's cultivation of physical health becomes an effective line of defense against forces that attempt to derail her story. Once it is taken away, as we see when she arrives at Moor House, she cedes control over her story. Until then, Jane aligns herself and her narrative with physical wellness.

Jane hints at the possible division between physical and emotional dangers when she states, in her capacity as retrospective narrator, that "[n]o severe or prolonged *bodily* illness followed this incident of the red-room: it only gave my nerves a shock, of which I feel the reverberations to this day" (25, emphasis added). Even when she admits to having "felt physically weak and broken down," she clarifies that "[her] worse ailment was an unutterable wretchedness of mind" (25). By creating, if not a firm separation between the body and the mind, a possible fissure between the two—such that if one fails the other might remain intact—Jane indicates the narrative value of temporarily separating physical disease from mental dis-ease.[32] For although medical discourse typically understood nervous shock as a physical problem (involving the nervous system), Jane's qualification ("only") suggests that "nerves," which she aligns with emotional fright, might be productively isolated from other forms of "bodily illness."[33] Jane's story, therefore, demonstrates an increasingly nuanced way of depicting and imagining the complex relationship between mental and physical health.

Her dependence on physical health is particularly evident at Lowood, a place permeated with disease and dis-ease. Alan Bewell has argued in "*Jane Eyre* and Victorian Medical Geography" that Brontë's depictions of Lowood engage directly in the public health debates of the period: "Brontë sets medicine against aesthetics, asking us to read the physical surrounding of Lowood the same way as doctors were being taught to read it, as a 'disease landscape.'"[34] Indeed, the atrocities at Lowood and the subsequent reforms they prompt speak to the larger politics of the novel. But while the girls' frozen limbs and their starvation and humiliation, as well as the typhus that kills them and the tuberculosis that eventually kills Helen Burns, dominate Jane's description of that period in her life, Lowood is not strictly or even primarily a scene of bodily illness. Rather, it functions for Jane as an affirmation of her relative good health—she never gets sick there, at least not seriously so. The chilblains and inflamed feet she endures are part of a collective experience rather a personal illness narrative—she refers to "our" insufficient clothing, "our shoes," and "our ungloved hands," using the specifics of her own condition, which begin as "a distracting irritation" and result in "torture," as representative of a larger problem (71).[35]

As with the oppositional strategies she has relied on for self-definition at Gateshead ("I was a discord," "a heterogeneous thing"), Jane's tendency to see herself in contrast to others and as an absence ("I was like nobody") becomes more explicit in her relationship with Helen Burns. Awed by Helen's patience and spirituality,

Jane realizes that she cannot subscribe to the same "doctrine of endurance" (67). When she feels the "impulse of fury against Reed, Brocklehurst, and Co.," she is prompted to assert, "I was no Helen Burns" (78). Jane's endurance is decidedly physical, and her foresight and imagination, unlike Helen's, are emphatically earthbound. Her claim of what she is not, though it refers specifically to Helen's lack of outrage when she is treated so poorly, is set in the context of health. As Helen reassures Jane that Brocklehurst's condemnation has likely helped rather than hurt Jane in the eyes of the other girls, Jane begins to notice that Helen is physically ill. Helen's quickened breathing and "short cough" make Jane "forget [her] own sorrows to yield to a vague concern" for Helen (83); these symptom also elucidate another important way in which Jane is "no Helen Burns"—she is not sick.

Not only does Jane not get sick and die but also she emerges from the typhus outbreak that devastates the school with a consciousness of her fortitude. In the midst of disease, Jane turns, as do medical definitions of health, to comparison rather than negation as a way to affirm the rarity and uniqueness of her condition:

> While disease had thus become an inhabitant of Lowood, and death its frequent visitor; while there was gloom and fear within its walls; while its rooms and passages steamed with hospital smells, the drug and the pastille striving vainly to overcome the effluvia of mortality, that bright May shone unclouded over the bold hills and beautiful woodland out of doors. Its gardens, too, glowed with flowers: hollyhocks had sprung up tall as trees, lilies had opened, tulips and roses were in bloom; the borders of the little beds were gay with pink thrift and crimson double daisies; the sweetbriars gave out, morning and evening, their scent of spice and apples; and these fragrant treasures were all useless for most of the inmates of Lowood, except to furnish now and then a handful of herbs and blossoms to put in a coffin.
>
> But I, and the rest who continued well, enjoyed fully the beauties of the scene, and season. (92)

Initially, disease and death appear to be the focus of this paragraph and certainly the focus of Jane's attention—an illness narrative of the first degree. But the fact of disease is subordinated to the vitality of the spring day. Jane begins "While disease" and therefore prepares the reader for something other than disease—its opposite. She delays the subject of the passage by repeating this subordination ("while") to highlight the "gloom" and "hospital smells"—all the by-products of illness—before reaching her main point: it was "bright May." Her turn to the freshness and health associated with spring—to the flowers in "bloom"—relieves us from the smells of death. Jane thus juxtaposes death/disease and life/health rhetorically (as the gloom/bloom rhyme bears out) and imagistically by substituting the "effluvia" for the "fragrant treasures" of spring. These "treasures" were, as she explains, "useless" to the sick girls, and while Jane's telling bears witness to the tragedy of Lowood, it is not her sole or even guiding purpose. Jane begins the subsequent paragraph "But I," thus asserting her condition as part of the minority experience—"forty-five of the eighty girls lay ill"—at the same time identifying herself as different even from "the rest" who are also healthy (90). This "I" is decidedly "well" and "enjoy[ing] fully the beauties of the scene, and season." Jane reflects not only the pleasures that come with being in good health but also the significance of defining and sustaining health to the production of her story.

Indeed, Jane suspends the story of her time at Lowood, "pass[ing] over a space of eight years almost in silence" once the "unhealthy nature of the site" gets revealed and individuals who are more "benevolent" than Mr. Brocklehurst take charge (99). A therapeutic reading would highlight the importance of illness to this narrative lapse; once the threat is gone or cured and health is restored, Jane has no story to tell. A hygienic reading does not deny the role that disease plays but seeks to emphasize instead the significance of Jane's maintained health and her narrative's impulse to define it, in this case, against disease. Once it is removed, the threat to Jane's health no longer functions as a sign of her uniqueness, and she ceases to possess the necessary framework she has been using to define who she is. Her ambivalence about her circumstances at Lowood and her desire for "change," for a "new servitude," signify this lack (102). Not until she moves to a new situation and location can she renew the impulse to "keep in good health."

The repetition—the routine and the effort—of maintenance, rather than the rupture inherent to crisis, organizes Jane's story. Once again, health becomes a way for Jane to ground her story; she develops her health sense in response to the locations she inhabits or imagines and the people she encounters.[36] In each environment and with each personal connection, her struggle to maintain and thus know her health, and the preventionist tactics such preservation demands, competes with the more alluring (and inevitable) crisis that comes from illness and dis-ease. After Jane arrives at Thornfield, she explains that her "bodily health improved" and that she "gathered flesh and strength" (172). But before we give Thornfield the credit for her presumed "improvement," we must remember that Jane has a unique capacity to survive what most others cannot.[37] When Jane tells Rochester that she lived at Lowood school for eight years, he responds with incredulity: "Eight years! You must be tenacious for life. I thought half the time in such a place would have done up any constitution! No wonder you have rather the look of another world" (143). Rochester's need to interpret Jane's strength as the stuff of fairy tales—in addition to being part of their bizarre flirtation ritual—reinforces and accentuates Jane's tendency to depict herself as unique and peculiar. Rochester's diagnosis of Jane turns to the metaphorical, as he imagines her, contra Brocklehurst, as having a "clean conscience" and "unpolluted memory . . . without blot or contamination." Jane is an ideal, an absence (she is "clean," "unpolluted"). While she still uses negation and comparison (she is no Blanche Ingram, either) to define herself, she also begins to see herself as Rochester does, "a rara avis," a salubrious fiction, and the "instrument of [his] cure" (253).

Thornfield is, as critics have noted, a site of serious illness. And, indeed, Bertha Mason's insanity has drawn significant critical attention.[38] Although I have bracketed the role that psychological health plays in Jane's narrative, I want to turn briefly to the tension between psychological and physical health and to the impossibility of preserving *mens sana in corpore sano* at Thornfield. Brontë provides chilling examples of psychological turmoil and psychosexual drama, not only through Rochester's sadistic wooing practices but also through Bertha Mason's history, behavior, and treatment. Significantly, though, it is only as an act of desperation that Rochester attempts to deny Jane the distinction of being "a rara avis" and to retract his claims about her wellness. When Jane tells Rochester about her encounter with a strange being, whom he knows to be Bertha, he turns to the language of medicine, diagnosing her as "hypochondriacal" and suffering from "mental terrors" (328), a label that, although she has used it on herself, she refuses to accept. The more she tells the story of Bertha donning and then trampling her wedding veil, and the more Rochester refuses Jane's version of herself, the more certain she becomes of her own condition. She concludes her tale by noting, "I lost consciousness . . . from terror"; she asserts that though "enfeebled, [she] was not ill." She follows this assertion with the demand that Rochester tell her "who and what that woman was" (327). Jane refuses to allow Rochester to brand her nerves as weak. Not until the next day, when Bertha's identity as Rochester's wife becomes known, does Jane define herself as "insane" but determined to "hold to the principles received by [her] when [she] was sane" (365). When she believes herself to be in bad or questionable (mental) health, she turns to her physical health, relying on it to help her escape becoming yet another one of Rochester's mistresses.

Jane's exodus from Thornfield is both a return to and an enactment of the Brocklehurst encounter with which I began. Having fled the drama of Thornfield, she reaffirms her initial investment in bodily health. When Jane reaches Moor House, however, the authority to define her health gets transferred temporarily to St. John—although, of course, as the narrator/author of her autobiography, Jane Rochester maintains ultimate control. St. John is among the few (men) to interpret Jane as healthy, and when he saves her from dying on his doorstep, he expresses little concern about her distress, repeatedly undercutting the therapeutic narrative into which she has cast herself. Rather than rushing to Jane's aid, he hangs back to eavesdrop on Hannah, who refuses Jane's appeal for help. He steps in only after Jane proclaims, "I can but die" (386). Only then does he conclude, with scientific objectivity, that Jane's "is a peculiar case" and that he "must examine into it"; he commands her to "rise, and pass before [him] into the house." When one of the women asks, "Is she ill, or only famished?" St. John's answer not only determines the course of treatment but also establishes the terms by which she may claim health. To be "only" famished is not to be ill in the sense of suffering from a disease. Indeed, during her recovery, St. John asserts that her "state of lethargy was the result of reaction from excessive and protracted fatigue," and he "pronounced it needless to send for a doctor: nature, he was sure, would manage best, left to herself. . . . There was no disease" (390). While Jane is decidedly not healthy by Johnson's terms ("free from bodily pain and sickness"), she is also not quite ill. St. John reads her condition comparatively, as falling somewhere below the average but still along the continuum of health.

St. John's desire to keep Jane well—or, more precisely, his impulse to read her as healthy rather than diseased—becomes a defining feature of their relationship. During her convalescence, and before she tells the story of how she came to arrive at the Rivers' doorstep, Jane overhears Diana chide St. John for claiming that Jane "looks sensible, but not at all handsome." Diana implies that it would not be accurate to judge Jane's appearance, since "[s]he is so ill." St. John's response that "ill or well, she's always plain" confirms what Jane has always said about herself (she is plain), but it also conflates illness and health by tacitly denying illness the capacity to alter Jane in any fundamental way. By constructing Jane as not only healthy but also, in effect, immune to illness, St. John creates for himself the perfect missionary wife. And while his early assessment of Jane anticipates his plan, it is not until after Jane becomes an heiress and attempts to regain control of her story that St. John's assertions about her health become more emphatic. When Mary and Diana urge Jane to forgo her weekly visit to Morton school during inclement weather, St. John claims, "Jane is not such a weakling as you would make her . . . she can bear a mountain blast, or a shower, or a few flakes of snow, as well as any of us." And as if consulting medical advice, he echoes Rochester's earlier claim: "Her constitution is both sound and elastic;—better calculated to endure variations of climate than many more robust" (458). Jane's constitution is not only "sound" but also better than most; it is unique and rare, a quality that suits his needs and has, until now, suited her own.

When Jane contemplates St. John's loveless marriage proposal, she returns to her best weapon: her health. And in so doing she regains control of her story. Jane acknowledges that it is in her power to assent to his will but that doing so would mean death. She recalls thinking, "'I *can* do what he wants me to do: I am forced to see and acknowledge that,'—I meditated—'that is, if life be spared me. But I feel mine is not an existence to be long protracted under Indian sun'" (466). Significantly, only after "meditat[ing]" does Jane find a solution to her problem—she is physically unfit for the climate of the Indian subcontinent. We see Jane's mind at work here, searching for a way out but not quite certain until she recalls in midthought, as signified by the dashes and the repetition of "that," that she can claim her desire to "keep in good health, and not die." Diana concurs: "You would not live three months there, I am certain" (478)—this assessment of a woman who has survived multiple exposures to typhus and will live out the rest of her days at Ferndean Manor, a place not fit to let or even to house a madwoman. The assumption that Jane would certainly die in India but could live (thrive, even) in a "dank" and remote house in England is not surprising (497). As the medical advice of the time warns, the English constitution was not suited to the subcontinent's climate. Critics have demonstrated how such a "fact" was often used as proof of English health. William Strange notes, however, that the body can adapt to various circumstances. And, indeed, Jane's preventive tactics—her refusal to be Rochester's mistress or St. John's wife—are part of what sustain her health and, at least metaphorically, keep her out of at least one fiery climate: the "hell" of impetuous feeling and passion that Reverend Brocklehurst ominously declared to be her fate.

Jane has managed to avoid that particular pit throughout her narrative, so it is fitting that she should return to Rochester on a cold and rainy evening and to a house overgrown with foliage, "scarce[ly] . . . distinguishable from the trees" (497).[39] She finds Rochester maimed and partially blind and offers herself as the cure he predicted she would be.[40] With the help of "an eminent oculist," he "recover[s] the sight of [his] one eye" (520). But Rochester's health is none of our concern. He need only be healthy enough to become a father. Jane, in contrast, has been protecting and proving her good health all along, which at Ferndean means not only caring for Rochester but also bearing his children. She speaks of their "first born," implying that others follow, but does not dwell on her own fertility or deliveries. Instead, she turns to death and to one who could not keep in good health.

St. John Rivers dies in India, "anticipat[ing] his sure reward, his incorruptible crown" (521). Here Jane revises her answer to Brocklehurst, but only slightly. There are, in fact, two ways to keep out of hell—one is to not die, and the other is to sacrifice oneself to heaven. Unlike Brontë's contemporaries who criticized the novel for its religious irreverence,[41] Stevie Davies suggests in his introduction to *Jane Eyre* that the ending "treads a path of ambivalent Christian heresy and transgressive traditionalism: it prefers the symbol (human marriage) over the thing symbolized (union with Christ)."[42] Perhaps even more than any union, symbolic or otherwise, the end reflects Jane's preference for health, for knowing "what it is" and determining to keep it. Reading for health is less about finding a cure or the happy ending, less about "plain Jane's progress" or even the final "reward," and more about the vigilance and self-assessment that go into the maintenance of such stories.

Two

Isolation

Chapter Three

Quarantine, Social Theory, and *Little Dorrit*

Health in Charles Dickens's novels is precarious: it is always threatened, often absent, and only occasionally recoverable. Above all, health for Dickens was a matter of public interest. By the middle of the nineteenth century, debates about how best to manage and maintain the public's health had taken center stage, focusing largely on the most effective method for preventing the spread of epidemic diseases. Following the advice of lead sanitationists Thomas Southwood Smith and Edwin Chadwick, Dickens lent his voice and popularity to the sanitary cause, arguing that clean, dry, airy, spacious environments were the key not only to public safety but also to defining and preserving public health.[1] As he explains in an early preface to *Martin Chuzzlewit* (1849, 1850): "In all my writings, I hope I have taken every available opportunity of showing the want of sanitary improvements in the neglected dwellings of the poor."[2] So adept was Dickens at depicting these diseases of neglect that, as Janis McLarren Caldwell notes, "Victorian medics were largely enthusiastic readers of Dickens. Medical journals not infrequently carried articles on Dickens adjacent to articles on pathology and diagnostics."[3] *Little Dorrit* (1857),[4] like all of Dickens's other works, features its share of slums and wretches: from Amy Dorrit's fly-infested birthplace and the Clennams' decrepit house to the suicidal Mr. Merdle and the recalcitrant Tattycoram, medical and metaphorical illnesses abound, and some form of treatment seems in order.

But as I have been suggesting, reading only for diseases and their cures obscures the complex ways that health, and the narrative structures that define it, operates in fiction and in the culture more broadly. Dickens's novels, like Austen's, interweave hygienic and therapeutic narratives, turning to prevention as a way to imagine complicated social interactions. Whereas Austen's works supplement professional advice, teaching readers about the intricate temporal aspects of preventionist thinking, Dickens's narratives offer limited guidance, often undercutting prevailing wisdom and even ignoring his political agenda. Filthy air and tainted people pervade *Little Dorrit* and align with Dickens's sanitationist allegiances,[5] but the uncertainty and necessary risk associated with the competing form of prevention—quarantine—are what come to matter most. For rather than dismiss quarantine as an outmoded and dangerous method of prevention, as any good sanitary reformer might (as Southwood Smith does in the Board of Health's *Report on Quarantine* [1849]),[6] Dickens instead turns to it in *Little Dorrit*, finding it curiously beneficial and unexpectedly salubrious. Quarantine reflects the contradiction and confusion that permeate the social world Dickens observes and creates. By centering on bodies in quarantine and anxieties about physical touch, Dickens presents readers with an alternative model of a healthy community, one that imagines the need for a delimited space that simultaneously protects and endangers—and thus binds together—the lives of its inhabitants.

Dickens invokes this paradox in book 1, chapter 2, first by highlighting the hazards of quarantine and then by demonstrating its benefits. We meet the novel's hero, Arthur Clennam, in quarantine talking to his new friend, the "comely and healthy" Mr. Meagles, who cannot help but ask, "What have we ever been in for?" Arthur's answer, which he admits is "no very strong reason," adheres to public health policy: "[W]e come from the East, and as the East is the country of the plague—" (30). By 1856–57, the period during which *Little Dorrit* was serialized, Britain had been devastated by two cholera outbreaks, and a third was on its way.[7] Despite Mr. Meagles's comical complaints, anxieties about epidemic diseases were real, and debates over how to prevent their spread persisted throughout much of the century. Mr. Meagles interrupts Arthur's half-hearted justification, claiming, "I have had the plague continually, ever since I have been here, I am like a sane man shut up in a madhouse; I can't stand the suspicion of the thing. I came here as well as ever I was in my life; but to suspect me of the plague is to give me the plague. And I have had it—and I have got it" (30). As the repetition of "I" in his diatribe suggests, Meagles objects on personal grounds, demonstrating little interest in the utilitarian wisdom offered in *The Lancet* (1837) that while "there can only be one sentiment respecting the hardship which [quarantine laws] impose upon the uninfected coming from infected places, the good of the few must yield to the benefit of the many" (72).

Hepworth Dixon remarks on this problem rather glibly in an early review of *Little Dorrit,* noting, "In a prison, you may, perhaps, catch a fever and die. In quarantine you are pretty certain to do so."[8] This criticism was axiomatic and addresses quarantine's central paradox: instead of preventing disease, quarantine may actually cause it.[9] But Dixon also admits that *Little Dorrit* captures "[s]ome of the beauties of this sort of civilized confinement."[10] Rather than totally barring contact, quarantine limits and "civilizes" it, providing a method for arranging and managing social interactions. Indeed, as Meagles claims later in the novel, quarantine was such "an uncommonly pleasant thing," he "often wished [him]self back again" (209). Thus, while we might agree with Meagles about the absurdity of being locked up, we recognize the fundamental value of this form of prevention and this model of health for Dickens: the "few" who are confined—like Arthur and Mr. Meagles—are not alone; they are very much together. Quarantine functions as more than a convenient setting for introducing characters and more than a metaphor for their thwarted and restricted lives.[11] It produces the narrative it is designed to prevent, asking us to become aware of who is touching whom, what that might mean, and how such contact links these characters' plots. The sustained isolation and delimited contact that result from quarantine create and fortify the community, providing time and space for characters to connect their stories, as they tell and embody their cautionary tales. This model of sociability preserves and defines the health not only of individuals but also—ultimately (and ideally)—of the nation.

By turning to quarantine, a system designed to keep people apart while forcing them into even closer contact, Dickens constructs a world—a realist fiction—in *Little Dorrit* about socially hopeful, if potentially perilous, contact, something he explored ten years earlier in *Pictures from Italy* (1846).[12] A brief anecdote, which takes up only a few pages of Dickens's travel narrative, speaks not about the politics of quarantine but about two characters whose relationship captures his imagination and expresses the physical touch that makes quarantine such a risky *and* delightful place.[13] Initially distraught about being detained—arguing, as Meagles might, that there was "nothing whatever the matter all the time"—Dickens makes the most of his isolation by hosting an impromptu party (*Pictures*, 76). When Dickens's tour guide procures (of his own volition) "a wicker basket, folded in linen cloth; . . . [with] two great bottles of wine, a roast fowl, some salt fish chopped with garlic, a great loaf of bread, a dozen or so peaches, and a few other trifles, . . . the whole party on board were made merry" (77). Two figures in particular stand out in Dickens's account of the quarantine party: the "little loquacious Frenchman," "who had got drunk in five minutes," and the Cappuccino Friar, "who had taken everybody's fancy mightily and was one of the best friars in the world" (77). Dickens becomes the omniscient narrator and observes and comments on these two men, explaining to his readers how the Frenchman took an especial interest in the Friar, such as "a mouse might bestow on a lion," "occasionally [rising] on tiptoe to slap the Friar on the back" (78). The Friar, though less invested in the friendship than the Frenchman, embraces the sociability of the moment—"laughing lustily from pure good-humour" (79). Isolation and closeness and the slap-on-the-back camaraderie depicted here foster not disease and death but healthy connections.[14] In the end, the friar and the Frenchman go their separate ways, but the moment of sociability lives on in Dickens's narrative. Individuals are connected medically through a desire to preserve health in this vignette, and public health policy is what imposes these connections.

THE DEBATE: PEOPLE VERSUS PLACES

Quarantine was not always or even generally thought of as a civilizing force. Critics and proponents alike agreed that it interfered with commerce, obstructed personal freedom, and put people at greater risk for catching disease.[15] What they could not agree on was the extent to which quarantine stopped the spread of epidemics. They could not, therefore, agree to abolish it completely; something about quarantine made sense. The problem, of course, was that disease transmission remained largely a mystery through much of the nineteenth century, although some, such as Thomas Southwood Smith, were unequivocal about the right method of prevention. In the *Report on Quarantine* (1849), Southwood Smith offers anecdotal and fictional evidence to support his claims about the threat that quarantine, and the theory of contagion on which it was founded, posed to sanitary reform.[16] He declares, "To assume the propagation by touch [that is, contagion] whether by the person or of the infected articles, and to overlook that by corruption of the air, is at once to increase the real danger, from exposure to noxious effluvia, and to divert attention from the true means of remedy and prevention" (47).[17]

The word *contagion*, etymologically related to *contact* (*con* 'together' and *tangĕre* 'to touch'), gets transformed in Smith's narrative to the more personal term *touch*, and because "air," not "touch," spreads disease, sanitary reform, not quarantine, must be the only "true" remedy. Of course, even contagionists recognized that the air acted as a vehicle for the spread of disease; if you were close enough to the person, you might not have to touch him in order to get infected by the emanations from his body. Southwood Smith, however, was intent on keeping the two theories about health (rhetorically) separate to focus on the absurdity of fearing touch—or, rather, the absurdity of fearing touch for the wrong reasons.

When he proceeds to illustrate why touch cannot possibly account for the transmission of epidemic disease, Smith creates, as a novelist might, a fantastic fiction: "According to the hypothesis of contagion, no matter how pure the air, no matter what the condition of the fever ward, if the physician only feels the pulse of the patient, or touches him with the sleeve of his coat, though he may not catch the disease himself, he may communicate it by a shake of the hand to the next friend he meets; or that friend, without catching it himself, may give it to another; or if the physician wash and fumigate his hand, but neglect the cuff of his coat, he may still convey the deadly poison to every patient whose pulse he feels during the day" (*Report*, 47). This transmission narrative features a doctor-hero who must be fearful of physical contact with his patient, as the basic job of taking a pulse or a chance brush of the sleeve could unleash an epidemic.[18] The patient's body may be the host of the disease, but the physician is responsible for spreading it through a basic form of sociable human interaction: shaking hands with a friend. Smith presents the fallout from this fictional contagion story as the inability to touch one another, to even touch a friend. He applies this paranoid scenario to the quarantine experience to demonstrate how we must *not* think about epidemic disease. Here, quarantine becomes a metonym for touch—and to discredit it, he must rule out touch as a problem.[19] In constructing this alarmist, absurdist story, Smith undermines quarantine while transforming it into a narrative about speculation, suspicion, and, most of all, contact between fictional people.

Dickens's speech to the Metropolitan Sanitary Society (1851) offers a similarly paranoid version of preventive—hygienic—thinking about anticipated transmission. Rather than showing why contact is absurd, however, Dickens demonstrates the dangers of filth and air: "[T]hat no one can estimate the amount of mischief which is grown in dirt; that no one can say, here it stops, or there it stops, either in its physical or its moral results, . . . is now as certain as it is that the air from Gin Lane will be carried, when the wind is Easterly, into May Fair."[20] This narrative of hazardous emanations (miasma) reads like the speculation Smith offers in his apocalyptic contagion narrative: the doctor checks a pulse, shakes a hand, touches a cuff, and wreaks havoc.[21] But even as Smith assured his readers in 1825, "Epidemic disease is not contagious because the human race continues to exist,"[22] the "truth" is that even by the 1850s no one knew precisely what caused or spread epidemic disease.

The world before germ theory—the world of Smith and of *Little Dorrit*—though largely lost to us now, was oddly confused and intensely scrutinized. People could see (or smell) that diseases moved, but nobody could see *how* disease moved. John Snow's discovery that cholera was transmitted by a contaminated water supply during the 1854 outbreak would alter the topography of disease awareness, but not for a while. His theory did not curry favor among powerful sanitationists and, therefore, was not accepted as conclusive until the subsequent epidemic in 1866. Even then, sanitationists found a way to hold strong to their theory of transmission. Part of the problem was that Snow did not know precisely what caused the contamination. As Steven Johnson explains in *The Ghost Map* (2006), "Cholera, Snow argued, was caused by some as-yet-unidentified agent that victims ingested, either through direct contact with the waste matter of other sufferers, or, more likely, through drinking water that had been contaminated with that waste. Cholera was contagious, yes, but not in the way small pox was contagious. Sanitary conditions were crucial to fighting disease, but foul air had nothing to do with its transmission."[23] More than presenting an illness narrative on a grand scale, Johnson's study reveals how Snow's work on public health benefited from the sociability of the curate Henry Whitehead, whose "local knowledge" of the people and their interactions would aid his developing theory.[24] Whitehead located the "index case" (the initial cause of the infection), which allowed Snow to determine the route of transmission through the Broad Street pump.

Until bacteriology was fully accepted,[25] which would not happen until the end of the century, the best anyone could do was to think in terms of people and places and to understand prevention and thus health as isolation or sanitation or some combination of the two.[26] Although contagionists and anticontagionists were both "influential," they were still "very much in the minority. . . . The bulk of contemporary opinion preferred to consider each disease in the 'epidemic, endemic and contagious' category individually and specifically, and to see 'doubtful' diseases [plague, yellow fever, continued fever, influenza, and cholera] as contingently contagious."[27] George Rosen explains that "limited or contingent contagion [attempted] to conciliate or compromise the miasmatic [anticontagionist/sanitationist] and contagionist theories."[28] In this view—one that Smith never specifically mentions—many believed that "infections were caused by contagion, but only arose if other elements existed such as appropriate atmospheric conditions."[29] Though they accommodated both theories, of miasma and of contagion, "limited contagionists" sided with miasmatists when it came to preventive measures, "tend[ing] to concentrate on cleaning up the environment and providing proper drainage, rather than on isolation or quarantine procedures."[30]

Thus, while Dickens was writing *Little Dorrit,* the questions remained: Did epidemics spread through contact between people (were they contagious) or through the noxious atmosphere (were they miasmic)? Or was it a combination of both? If they were contagious, then isolating people should stop the spread; if it was the air, then quarantine would not only fail but also re-create the unsanitary conditions that cause disease in the first place. The answer to how epidemic diseases were spread would determine the most effective means of prevention: Was it quarantine or sanitation? Was it both—or something else entirely?[31] The successful preventionist strategy would teach people better ways to preserve and define health. Determining a winner was not easy, but this indeterminacy is precisely what contributes to Dickens's social theory and sense of community in *Little Dorrit*.

While the public-speaking Dickens was concerned with the dangers of "vitiated air" and putrefaction and believed in the sanitary cause, the novelist Dickens found value in the opposing view provided by quarantine. The moments of touch (or its refusal) and the paranoia that shapes these encounters in quarantine are central to the sociability that is so important to his novels and his politics. That Dickens is not bound by the distinctions among the various theories of transmission is evident.[32] That his novels and his conception of health rely on maintaining the uncertainty surrounding the preventive measures defining these theories is, perhaps, less so. *Bleak House* (1853),[33] for example, is arguably Dickens's most famous fictional appeal on behalf of the sanitary idea. It also, however, reflects this ambivalence about disease transmission and about the measures one must take to preserve and define health.[34]

When Jo the crossing-sweeper carries an unnamed illness from the city to the country and transmits it to Esther Summerson through her maid Charley, the illness unites plots as much as it critiques public policy.[35] As critics (and the novel itself) have observed, the spread of disease from the London slums to Bleak House becomes the primary link between classes and represents the physical and social disease plaguing British society.[36] But within this push for sanitary reform lies a social and narrative theory that turns to contagion and quarantine and thus bumps up against Dickens's political views about sanitation. What is also significant about the care Jo receives is the way it reflects each character's personal response to the sick body. The fog may be everywhere, and the city may need a good moral and medical scrubbing, but the fact remains that Jo transmits his disease to Esther through direct contact with Charley. And although the decaying houses of Tom-All-Alone's and the decomposing bodies of the burial grounds are largely responsible for Jo's illness (in no small part because they represent society's inattentiveness to the basic needs of the poor), it is touch that communicates disease.[37] Only Skimpole, who "retreat[s] . . . to the drawing room," registers the dangers of physical contact with Jo (493). The rest fear for the boy's well-being and demonstrate their lack of concern about their own health by bringing him into their home, standing next to him and caressing him, touching and carrying him. Jarndyce, Esther, Charley, and the servants at Bleak House seem—despite Skimpole's prophetic warning—to take no precautions against possible infectious touch. (Ada is significantly absent with a cold.)

And why should they? Not everyone with whom he comes into contact becomes ill. Jarndyce willingly and without fear "touch[es] him and examin[es] his eyes" before deciding to keep him in the "wholesome" stable loft (493). As in Smith's doctor-narrative, only some of the people get sick. Esther even finds pleasure in the sight of Jo bundled in the arms of the servants who carry him to the loft and call him "Old Chap" (496). Dickens offers a positive—healthy—version of contagion, one that Thomas Carlyle invoked ten years earlier in *Past and Present* (1843) as a metaphor for reform, which he argued must "radiate outwards [from home] irrepressible, into all that we touch and handle, speak and work; kindling ever new light, by incalculable contagion, spreading in geometric ratio, far and wide—doing good only, wheresoever it spreads, and not evil."[38] The metaphorical contagion in this scenario creates social health, and the "incalculable" that Carlyle embraces must not be quarantined—contact is, as Smith imagines it, unlimited and uncontrolled. Contagion for Carlyle is more than a metaphor; it is a medical reality that literally connects us. In the story of an Irish widow suffering from typhus whom nobody will help, Carlyle argues: "Nothing is left but that she prove her sisterhood by dying, and infecting you with typhus. Seventeen of you lying dead will not deny such proof that she was flesh of your flesh; and perhaps some of the living may lay it to heart."[39] As Tina Young Choi points out, "The inevitability of biological connection finally and ironically becomes that which re-cements social connection in the urban environment."[40]

This generative version of contagion operates similarly in *Bleak House*—although, unlike Carlyle, Dickens does not let it go unchecked. Quarantine's capacity to delimit contact becomes important to Dickens's vision of how contagion produces narrative, how it generates a humane and thus healthy society. Esther's quick thinking contains the disease, preventing its spread beyond her cordon sanitaire. The shift from miasma to contagion, from sanitation (Tom-All-Alone's) to quarantine (Esther's isolation) is both a medical shift and an ethical and narratological one. Concern over the living conditions of the many becomes, here, concern about managing individual contact and intimacy among the few.[41] Contact both threatens lives and saves them, and our knowledge about disease transmission, no matter what we might like to believe, is always provisional, uncertain, and subject to contradiction. Being part of a community involves risk, and learning how best to navigate that risk is central to Dickens's conception of public health and to the plot in *Little Dorrit.*[42]

ARTHUR CLENNAM'S QUARANTINE NARRATIVE

Quarantine is a place where stories form and merge—a place where (to borrow from Carlyle) we have the opportunity to prove our humanity or reject it altogether. In *Little Dorrit,* Dickens uses this facet of quarantine to construct Arthur's story, shuttling him from one model of quarantine to another (Marseille, Miss Wade, Mrs. Clennam, Pancks, the Marshalsea), from one form of contact to another, to draw out and fortify his narrative, binding it to those around him. This process begins in book 1, chapter 2, where the intimacy created by quarantine is largely physical and (deliberately) dangerous. Imagining himself to be the evidence for the plague, Meagles argues that the "fellows" (that is, the officers of health) can only "mak[e] out their case" for declaring quarantine if they see signs of disease. To prove himself innocent, Meagles turns to his daughter, Pet, asking Arthur, "[S]imply as between man and man, you know, DID you ever hear of such damned nonsense as putting Pet in quarantine?" (31). We are left to assume that Mr. Meagles refers to her beauty, purity, and good manners as somehow rendering her immune to disease. By presenting Pet in this way, Mr. Meagles asks Arthur to become an expert—as we all should be—of health and to deem his daughter healthy, nonthreatening, and beyond suspicion. Meagles gives Arthur permission to admire Pet and to look at (though not necessarily touch) her body. And all Arthur can do when faced with this silly request is reply that Pet has "ma[de] even quarantine enjoyable" (31). As ridiculous as Mr. Meagles's logic might be (if his pretty young daughter is in quarantine, then something must be wrong with the system), such thinking allows him to take charge of the narrative and transform it from one about potential plague into one about family affection and romance.

While touch is a key element of quarantine, as Meagles makes clear in this moment, suspicion is equally treacherous—though to be suspicious in this context generally means fearing touch. Smith makes a similar point about the dangers of suspicion in his *Report on Quarantine*:[43] "[T]he invariable effect of quarantine as hitherto practiced in all countries has been the congregation and confinement of the sick and those who, though not actually sick, are suspected to have in them the seeds of disease . . . the congregation and confinement of such persons in limited space, and often in a filthy ship and an unhealthy locality, and always under circumstances calculated to excite apprehension and alarm."[44] As long as quarantine exists, Smith suggests, we will continue to need it, for it not only replicates the physical environment (the miasmas) that anticontagionists believed were responsible for disease but also generates the very psychological conditions—suspicion and apprehension—that intensify the potential physical threat. Mr. Meagles's claim that the real danger and fear associated with quarantine is "the suspicion of the thing" draws the same conclusion (with different evidence), implying that far from preventing anything, quarantine proliferates and exacerbates that which it is meant to obstruct. In quarantine, thought, not just touch, connects us, and as the narrative unfolds, suspicion and touch become a significant form of narrative transmission among characters. It motivates Arthur, terrifies Affery, and undoes Mr. Dorrit.

To align suspicion, paranoia, and touch and to reframe the role of prevention, Dickens constructs a modified crisis-cure narrative that is curiously free of medical diseases. He also removes from our consideration the overtly political public health agenda we encounter in *Bleak House*. The fear of epidemic disease and the call for prevention are not, as in *Bleak House*, predominantly literal. These absences reconfigure quarantine's affiliation with disease, opening space for the possibility of a healthy narrative formed through contagious contact. As the title of chapter 8 in book 2 ("The Progress of an Epidemic") suggests, the plague is entirely metaphorical, used to describe speculation mania and fallout from Mr. Merdle's fraudulent banking practices.[45] This episode exemplifies the flexibility Dickens saw in these theories of disease transmission and the structures of prevention that these theories produce.[46]

Although the plague was (according to proponents of quarantine) contagious—a problem of individual, personal contact[47]—Dickens initially dismantles the plague metaphor in this chapter by disconnecting it from any one body or any single instance of contact. The plague is in the air, and Dickens imagines disease as a narrative device designed to explain a social reality: "That it is at least as difficult to stay a moral infection as a physical one; that such a disease will spread with the malignity and rapidity of the Plague; that the contagion, when it has once made head, will spare no pursuit or condition, but will lay hold on people in the soundest health, and become developed in the most unlikely constitutions; is a fact as firmly established by experience as that we human creatures breathe an atmosphere" (597). The narrator's exaggerated rhetoric draws our attention away from any one body as the cause of disease, referring only to the bodies (multiple) of the formerly healthy who might suffer. For, although "the contagion" in this case originates with Merdle, it is not spread by contact with his person.[48] Rather, it is "the name of Merdle" that "fill[s] the air" and transmits disease. George Yeats observes in "'Dirty Air': *Little Dorrit*'s Atmosphere" that as Dickens "develops the conceit, [he] focuses less on the origin of sickness and more upon its transmission."[49] While Yeats's emphasis on transmission and his claim that the "air" is aligned with Merdle's nefarious business practices offer a useful way to read the plague imagery in this episode, the novel's investment in quarantine and in opposing modes of transmission suggests that "the contagion" also functions (perhaps simultaneously) as a simile to describe the ubiquity and anonymity of "disease." Thus, rather than endorse a single definition of public health, Dickens seems always to expose, even in the most miasmic moments of the novel, the instability of the theories that surround it.[50]

This tension between theories of transmission and the preventive tactics they represent becomes more evident as the narrator offers an isolationist solution to the problem rather than a sanitationist one. Readers are assured that it would be "[a] blessing beyond appreciation [that] would be conferred upon mankind, if the tainted, in whose weakness or wickedness these virulent disorders are bred, could instantly be seized and placed in close confinement (not to say summarily smothered) before the poison is communicable" (*Little Dorrit,* 597). The world of sanitary concerns, in which unsuspecting people become the victims of a bodiless force, gives way to the seizure, confinement, and extermination of individuals—"the tainted"—whose bodies, purposely or not, host the disease. This description of plague could have framed

Arthur's discussion with Mr. Meagles about the threat of a literal plague from book 1, chapter 2. But literal plagues and actual quarantines need not be feared.

This is particularly true for Arthur, who finds in quarantine friendship and family, the two things he needs most. Quarantine is a place where he can finally tell his story, which he has been keeping to himself his whole life.[51] As Arthur becomes a little lost in his admiration for Meagles's proof of health (his daughter, Pet), Mr. Meagles can only draw him back into conversation by "tapp[ing] him on the arm" (31), a physical reminder that Arthur has a place in this story and a job to do in the narrative. And while Meagles's detour into Pet's presumed health, which we learn later is not quite the whole story, fails to explain what Mr. Meagles has "got," it does begin to direct our attention to what Arthur has "got"—and must keep—and how we might read the quarantine experience as central to the production and maintenance of his story. Having lived in China for twenty years, Arthur has essentially been removed from society. He has been isolated, but not in the way quarantine isolates. He has nobody with whom to share his tale, certainly not the exotic "Chinese lad[ies]" Flora Finching imagines. Arthur meets the Meagles family while they are all touring in the East, but not until they are together in quarantine do they cultivate their lasting friendship. And it is not until the final hours of quarantine—the moment when they will be released from confinement and from each other—that Arthur first connects his story to someone else's. He asks Mr. Meagles if Pet has any siblings, a question that will allow Arthur to recall his own difficult upbringing. Pet's twin sister died as an infant, but the Meagleses, who were "not young" when they became parents, view the sisters as one: "When Pet has grown, that [dead] child has grown" (34), though how much she has been allowed to grow is questioned by their maid, Tattycoram, who complains that "they make a fool of [Pet], they spoil her" (42). As Mr. Meagles tells it, "Pet has always had a sort of grown-up life, though we have tried to adapt ourselves to her" (34). Whether her parents spoil her or are merely trying to adapt to her, they offer Pet the kind of familial love that Arthur hardly knows exists.

Although the content of the story is secondary to the fact that it gets told at all, it prompts Arthur to tell a similarly themed, though very different, tale. Like all prevention narratives, Arthur's story focuses on his desolate childhood. As an excuse for his lack of "will, purpose, hope," Arthur explains to his companion, "I am the son . . . of a hard father and mother. I am the only child of parents who weighed, measured, and priced everything: for whom what could not be weighed, measured and priced, had no existence" (35). But quarantine draws together two paradoxical narratives: Arthur's description of parental feeling and the story Mr. Meagles tells in which parents never cease to value a dead child and must continually adapt to the circumstances of the living one. Arthur and Mr. Meagles interweave their stories, and the process of anchoring Arthur, of giving his plot depth and purpose, begins here. Quarantine has achieved one of the two purposes for which it was designed (though not intended): after a period of sequestration, the "disease" expresses itself, gets contained, and is then transmitted. Dickens transforms quarantine from a public health nightmare into a model for health maintenance. Arthur's survival depends on developing "will, purpose, hope." As Sir John Sinclair notes in his *Code of Health*, "[w]hen the minds of persons have been fortified by hope, they either escape the contagion of any prevailing epidemic, or are infected by it in a milder manner than those are who give way to unfavorable apprehension."[52]

Quarantine's other job—the other way that it promotes healthy contact—is what public policy hopes it will do: isolate, obstruct, and terminate. We see this version of quarantine in the way that Dickens represents Miss Wade, one of the other "inmates." But in this case, unlike with Meagles, Dickens pathologizes quarantine. This is, as the narrator might say, "[h]ow not to do it"—a cautionary tale that aligns with Smith's extremist scenario. As if following strict laws of contagion, Miss Wade functions as a quarantine within quarantine, isolating herself and refusing, or at least resisting, touch—the "one medium of communication," according to *Fraser's Magazine* (1853),[53] that quarantine is designed to prevent. When Pet Meagles attempts to cultivate a relationship with Miss Wade, offering her father's assistance and "timidly touching her hand," Miss Wade rejects the offer both verbally and physically; under Pet's touch, Miss Wade's hand "lay impassive on the sofa between them" (39). When Mr. Meagles offers to shake her hand, the narrator explains, "[s]he would not have put out her hand, it seemed, but that Mr. Meagles put out his so straight before her, that she could not pass it. She put hers in it, and it lay there just as it had lain upon the couch" (39). This revulsion against touch, particularly after they have just been released from quarantine, represents a contagionist ethos that interprets contact between "persons" as undesirable and unhealthy.

Miss Wade shares her theory about contact by responding to Mr. Meagles's observation that they "may never meet again" with the following enigmatic statement: "In our course through life, we shall meet the people who are coming to meet *us*, from many strange places and many strange roads . . . and what is set to us to do to them, and what is set to them to do to us, will all be done"(39).[54] Miss Wade's warning draws together the two modes of transmission that define the quarantine debate: places and people. While places are part of Miss Wade's warning, they are not, despite their strangeness, our concern. The people are. The narrator repeats Miss Wade's premonitory statement at the end of the chapter: "And thus ever, by day and night, under the sun and under the stars, climbing the dusty hills and toiling along the weary plains, journeying by land and journeying by sea, coming and going so strangely, to meet and to act and react on one another, move all we restless travellers through the pilgrimage of life" (43). In this version, places (the "dusty hills," "weary plains," "land" and "sea") constitute the bulk of the description and seem to highlight the environment and the atmosphere as defining how the people will behave once they reach their destination. And yet by delaying the subject of this litany—we restless travelers—until the end of the sentence and the end of the chapter, Dickens underscores the novel's anticipation of people (plots) meeting and acting and reacting. Amanda Anderson observes that this "narrative revision" distances Miss Wade's "fatalis[m]" and "bitter[ness]" from the narrator's and the narrative's sense of contact by "stressing the universal weary struggle of life."[55] As Anderson notes, the narrator presents the "potentially interactive quality of social encounters."[56] I would add, too, that within the quarantine setting and in a novel that continually turns to the rhetoric of contagion and epidemic disease, acting and reacting exemplify a pathological sense of touch that Miss Wade represents and that the novel transforms into health through Arthur's story and particularly his contact with Amy Dorrit.

The sense of inevitable contact—and, as Miss Wade suggests, of doing to each other "what is set" to do—ultimately has less to do with location and everything to do with people and with questions about how to manage their contact and their stories. When Miss Wade sees Pet shrink from her vision, for "it implied that what was to be done was necessarily evil," Miss Wade reemphasizes her point by speaking directly to Pet: "You may be sure that there are men and women [who are] already on their road, who have their business with *you* and who will do it" (40). By representing contact as a mass of people—"men and women"—who are on their way, apparently, to trample Pet, Miss Wade implies that there is nothing anyone can do to stop it. She claims, in fact, that these various, unknown people "may be coming, for anything you know, or anything you can do to prevent it, from the vilest sweepings of this very town" (40). This warning marks a shift that is characteristic of Dickens's thinking on public health, a shift between the contagionist and miasmatist model of transmission, such that the people who come to "do evil" must come from somewhere ("the vilest sweepings"). But we are drawn back again to individuals and to the sense that while in quarantine Pet is safe from these encounters. For even Miss Wade, despite her interest in Pet, has not come to do her will. Rather, she has come to observe and to hate from a distance.

And this, for Dickens, is Miss Wade's problem: her impenetrability is a marker of her inhumanity. When Pet asks, "Are you . . . expecting any one to meet you here, Miss Wade," Miss Wade responds with a question: "I? No" (39). By her own philosophy, Miss Wade should know to expect someone to meet her somewhere, but in this instance her initial refusal to connect rhetorically (the "I?" response to a direct address, "Miss Wade," seems excessive) represents her desire to remain aloof from the party in general and from Pet in particular. We learn that Miss Wade "had either withdrawn herself from the rest or been avoided by the rest—nobody, herself excepted perhaps, could have quite decided which" (36). The narrator repeats this question just a few pages later: "[I]t would have been as difficult as ever to say, positively, whether she avoided the rest, or was avoided" (38). Within the context of quarantine, avoidance is protection, but the ambiguity evoked by the narrator's "perhaps" allows us to question this protective instinct and to remain suspicious of those who refuse touch.

Dickens further warns against the dangers of isolation without community through Miss Wade's curiosity about "the maid with the curious name" (40). After seeing Tatty in a fit for the third time, Miss Wade goads her into revealing what is wrong. Like Pet, Tatty is afraid of Miss Wade, but she is afraid for a very different reason. Tatty identifies Miss Wade with her "own anger, [her] own malice, [her] own—whatever it is." For her part, Miss Wade sees her own infected self in Tatty. The narrator explains that she "stood with her hand upon her bosom, looking at the girl, as one afflicted with a diseased part might curiously watch the dissection and exposition of an analogous case" (42). The accompanying illustration, entitled "Under the Microscope," depicts Miss Wade in such a stance, observing Tatty crouched on the floor with her head and arm partially covered by the coverlet. Although Miss Wade is in the position of observer, both women are, in effect, "under the microscope"; both are reduced to clinical cases. This pathological similarity between the two women draws Miss Wade to Tatty and becomes the driving metaphor for what the novel condemns as an unhealthy, because unproductive and sterile, form of contact. Here, the connection is figured less as contagion and more as chronic or hereditary—embedded in a character's temperament.

Not until Tatty involves Pet does a quarantine ethos emerge as protective and preventive. When Pet learns that Tatty has visited Miss Wade, Pet rejects Tatty's touch: "Take your hands away. I feel as if some one else is touching me!" (214). Pet reacts as a contagionist; but even more than fearing that Tatty has been tainted by her contact with Miss Wade, Pet imagines Tatty as embodying Miss Wade. Pet's only recourse is to refuse touch and to draw an imaginary boundary around her person. In an attempt to conciliate Tatty, Pet gives her hand back, explaining, "Miss Wade almost frightened me when we parted, and I scarcely liked to think of her just now as having been so near me without my knowing it" (214). While this nearness refers primarily to Miss Wade's presence on the property, Pet's "involuntary" withdrawal from Tatty speaks to the anxiety about how best to manage contact—both preventing it and permitting it—that structures the narrative encounters throughout the novel.[57]

Even for Miss Wade (and for Dickens), absolute isolation is impossible to sustain. Quarantine is, as Smith depicts it, a fiction or at least based on the fiction of contagion. It is permeable and faulty, and our need and compulsion to reach out physically to each other override even the strictest medical advice. Offering Arthur the letter of her life story is one of the only moments at which Miss Wade initiates "touch," literally and metaphorically extending her hand: "Shall I give you something I have written," she asks, "or shall I hold my hand?" (40). Arthur takes the letter and reads it, but her narrative stands alone, isolated from the novel's plot, never to become fully connected to it. The one time Miss Wade might link her story with Arthur's is to give Mr. Meagles the documents that Mrs.

Clennam's blackmailer, Rigaud, asks her to keep, but she refuses, and her story ends.

Arthur navigates both forms of quarantine—the isolationist version of Miss Wade and the sociable version represented by Meagles—throughout the novel. His first experience occurs when he returns to his mother's house in London, a place that bears a striking resemblance to quarantine but proves to draw too much from the contagionist model. The absence of touch creates an excess of suspicion, and Mrs. Clennam, the only other character in *Little Dorrit* to cultivate Miss Wade's form of physical and narrative isolation, equates quarantine with disease rather than with health. Her mode of prevention casts her as unhealthy and helps her to maintain this condition. The childhood tale Arthur told in quarantine has prepared us for Mrs. Clennam's aloofness. He described her as "strict," "stern," and "austere" and her religion as "a gloomy sacrifice of tastes and sympathies" (35). The road to this sterilized maternalism is paved with the metaphoric threat of disease. The narrator explains that "[i]n every thoroughfare, up almost every alley, and down almost every turning, some doleful bell was throbbing, jerking, tolling as if the Plague were in the city and the dead-carts were going round" (43). We are returned to the language of quarantine and to the place where the plague should have been stopped and where epidemic disease (at least as a simile) becomes the common marker against which all other desolation and despair must be measured.[58] And yet, as Arthur braces himself at a coffeehouse before going to see his mother for the first time in twenty years, this plague and the concern over contact/contagion attached to it transform into a filthy environment: "Fifty thousand lairs surrounded him where people lived unwholesomely, that fair water put into their crowded rooms on Saturday night, would be corrupt Sunday morning; albeit my lord, their country member, was amazed that they failed to sleep in company with their butcher's meat. Miles of close wells and pits of houses, where the inhabitants gasped for air, stretched far away towards every point of the compass. Through the heart of the town a deadly sewer ebbed and flowed in the place of a fine fresh river" (44). This language recalls the Dickens who gave speeches to the Metropolitan Sanitary Association, the Dickens who invented Tom-All-Alone's and Jacob's Island. Dickens "surround[s]" Arthur with the sanitary cause, a place where people "gas[p] for air" that has been tainted by slaughterhouse stench, a place where people are forced to smell and drink water tainted by "deadly" sewage. But he does not dwell there.

Mrs. Clennam's debilitated house and "airless room" at first fall under the umbrella of such unwholesome, miasmatic places (49). The "musty smell" and the impression of dirtiness Arthur finds in his room register the unhealthiness of the place of his childhood and seem to particularize and personalize the public health dangers and the "condition of England" we witnessed on his way there. Although a moral cleansing seems in order, this sanitary stance yields to the language of invalidism and inherited disease, and it concentrates our attention on the suspicious absence of maternal contact. When Arthur comments on the change in Mrs. Clennam's activities, she claims that a "rheumatic affection" and the "debility or nervous weakness" that comes with it prohibit her from leaving her room. Her "immovable face, as stiff as the folds of her stony head-dress," is mimicked by the "maimed table" and "crippled wardrobe" in Arthur's room. It is as if Mrs. Clennam has infected the furniture; objects that are by design immobile become even more so when imagined as extensions of her will. However, from the first, the invalid's investment in isolation and stasis takes on a contagious quality. She configures her room and her body as quarantine, limiting her physical contact with the outside world. She greets her son with "one glass kiss, and four stiff fingers muffled in worsted" (48–49). The narrator draws attention to the momentousness of this gesture by referring to it as an "embrace," as if to suggest that within Mrs. Clennam's world even the touch of four covered fingers counts as full physical contact (49).

And as we saw in quarantine, touch and suspicion are of a piece. After this initial visit with his mother, Arthur returns the following morning to question her about his father's dying actions: "'I want to ask you, mother, whether it ever occurred to you to suspect—'At the word Suspect, she turned her eyes momentarily upon her son, with a dark frown. . . . '—that he had any secret remembrance which caused him trouble of mind—remorse?'" (62).[59] This narratorial interruption, reminiscent of the way Meagles interrupted Arthur in quarantine, highlights suspicion and signifies what we will eventually learn about the hereditary "dis-ease" that afflicts the Clennam family: Mrs. Clennam is not Arthur's biological mother. As we learn later, Arthur's father had a child with another woman but, being too weak to resist, was forced into an unwanted marriage with the woman Arthur knows as his mother.

Before revealing Mrs. Clennam's secret and the truth of Arthur's story, Dickens enacts the Carlylean dictum (that we connect through disease) by turning to disease: Arthur must get sick. But while this moment seems ripe for a therapeutic reading about the hero's need for a cure, Dickens stages Arthur's infection within the paradoxical logic of quarantine, in which such transmissions do good instead of ill, in which curing is not the final goal. It is a moment of isolated intimacy that recalls the quarantine setting of chapter 2 and signifies Arthur's second significant encounter with post-Marseilles quarantine. This event is a modified version of the sociable contact he experienced with Meagles. Set in a cozy room with Mr. Pancks, pipes, and the Orient, "The Progress of an Epidemic" mimics the structure of contact we saw with Meagles and Arthur. Arthur invites one of his only friends, Pancks, to join him for dinner because, as Arthur explains it, "I am weary and out of sorts" (606); the longstanding struggle with the Circumlocution Office on behalf of his business partner and his recent encounter with Rigaud at his mother's house weigh "heavy on his lonely mind," and, by his own admission, he needs a trusted friend in whom he can confide (610). This affection, the narrator reminds us, developed as a result of Pancks's role in restoring the Dorrit fortune. After their dinner, Arthur offers Pancks his Eastern pipe, and the two friends discuss the wisdom of investing with Merdle. As Pancks assures Arthur that the investments are "safe and genuine," we enter the dangerous side of sociability. Pancks takes "as long a pull as his lungs would permit at his Eastern pipe, and look[s] sagaciously and steadily at Clennam while inhaling and exhaling too," and the narrator goes on to explain with some specificity that "[i]n those moments, Mr Pancks began to give out the dangerous infection with which he was laden. It is the manner of communicating these diseases; it is the subtle way in which they go about" (609). The dangerous infection is identified with the East and with person-to-person contact, but it also becomes part of the atmosphere, part of the vague and disembodied miasma that cannot be contained. The divisions (air, not touch, and cleanliness, not isolation), which are presumably essential to the management of public health, merge and dissolve in this moment. Neither theory applies. There is nothing to be done. The air (the smoke, the conversation, the trust) acts like touch, taking on the qualities of human contact. And the pipe, rather than functioning as a symbol of foreign contamination or an impersonal miasma, signifies male intimacy, comfort, and support—experiences the novel has endorsed throughout, despite its emphasis on Amy Dorrit's superior companionability.

Instead of condemning this friendship by depicting Pancks as the cause of disease or an extension of Merdle, Dickens binds these men through their circumstances and surroundings. The narrator argues that although the disease originated with "weakness and wickedness," it is not always transmitted by this same method: "Of whom Mr Pancks had taken the prevalent disease, he could no more have told than if he had unconsciously taken a fever. Bred at first, as many physical diseases are, in the wickedness of men, and then disseminated in their ignorance, these epidemics, after a period, get communicated to many sufferers who are neither ignorant nor wicked. Mr Pancks might, or might not, have caught the illness himself from a subject of this class; but, in this category he appeared before Clennam, and the infection he threw off was all the more virulent" (609–10). Dickens relies here, as he does elsewhere in his writing, not so much on what was known about the transmission of epidemic disease as on what was not known. The uncertainty about origins and etiology seems to make prevention a near impossibility; the recommended confinement and smothering we get at the beginning of the chapter lose some of their force. We do not know who (what "class" of person) originally infected Pancks. We do know that Pancks is responsible for "communicating" it to Clennam and that the scene of contagion stems from a single person, a fact that will weigh heavily on Pancks's heart and mind by the end of the novel. This description both accuses and exonerates Pancks; he is "neither ignorant nor wicked," and this, it seems, makes the infection more dangerous but also more hopeful than it might otherwise have been. The only way to protect Arthur, particularly in this vulnerable state, would have been to limit his personal contact with Pancks and thus deduct from his already limited domestic circle. In other words, the newly "infected" will become a healthier Arthur. As the dis-ease takes over his body, the chapter concludes as it began, as a medical guide to the diagnosis of disease: "[S]uch symptoms," the narrator explains, "when a disease of this kind is rife, are usually signs of sickening" (613). But this sickness does not need a cure. Rather, it represents a necessary condition that will make room for Amy Dorrit and will send Arthur into the isolated contact—the quarantine—he has needed and for which he has unconsciously been searching all along.

Arthur enters the narrative disconnected, detached, and uncertain; as he builds a chain of contact, we are reminded of his mother's refusal to touch. Mrs. Clennam's self-imposed isolation, effected though not demanded by her invalidism, does not, we learn, come from an innate or even cultivated abhorrence and fear of touch. It comes, rather, from a morality that requires a particular form of contact and from the disappointment of being rejected. She has been isolating herself and her story from virtually everyone around her, imagining that she could control and protect both, but as her narrative unfolds—as Rigaud forces her to tell it—she reveals that underlying her desire for complete isolation is a more tragic need for physical connection without suspicion.[60]

Although Arthur is not present during this third reenactment of quarantine, his story is nonetheless informed by his mother's experience, by a new form of contact that reveals her story, which comes before, or "prevents" (*præ* 'before' and *venīre* 'to come'), his own. Dickens depicts contact in the form of Rigaud's touch as central to her narrative and to its transmission. The scene, which parallels the one involving Pancks and Arthur, takes place in a space of intimacy and focuses on two individuals. But in this case, the touching is literal, and it signifies the simultaneous risks and benefits of delimited contact as opposed to absolute isolation. As the narrator explains it, Rigaud "leaned an arm upon the sofa close to her own, which he touched with his hand." He gives her arm a sinister tickle and then adopts the language of medicine, calling himself "something of a doctor" and asking her to "[l]et [him] touch [her] pulse." Even after she wrests her arm from his grip, he "tap[s] her arm, to beat his words home" (804). Rigaud uses touch as a way to activate the story about what he describes as "a strange marriage, and a strange mother, and a revenge, and a suppression" (804). This is not the first we have heard of Rigaud's hands, for his touch has been the focus of his own story. In book 1, chapter 1, for example, the narrator explains that his "hand . . . (seamed all over the back with ugly scratches newly healed) was unusually small and plump; would have been unusually white, but for the prison grime" (18). The scratches become part of the story of his wife's murder, a crime that "the law could not prove" he committed (143). This fixation on his hands persists, as when he is released from prison and we encounter him a second time at an inn, where the landlady, initially suspicious, sees that "he ha[s] a fine hand . . . and think[s] that he [is] not ill-looking after all" (143). Shortly after this reminder of his hands, he encounters his former cellmate at the same inn and commands him to "[t]ouch the hand of a gentleman!" (145).

Fully entrenched in the language of both models of disease transmission (miasma and contagion), Mrs. Clennam determines to speak and to tell her story to stop Rigaud from "taint[ing]" it with his "wickedness" (807). Her cautionary tale, which is told too late to do her any good, begins with a description of a tragic childhood. It is a story we have heard before from Arthur about his upbringing. Mrs. Clennam explains that she was "brought up strictly, and straitly. [Hers] was no light youth of sinful gaiety and pleasure. [Hers] were days of wholesome repression, punishment, and fear" (807). Her father assured her that young Clennam had experienced a similar upbringing and that he had "lived in a starved house, where rioting and gaiety were unknown, and where every day was a day of toil and trial like the last." Most important, however, she had been told, "his uncle's roof had been a sanctuary to him from the contagion of the irreligious and dissolute" (808). Though "contagion" here reads as a metaphor, it is for Mrs. Clennam very real—the evidence of which we can see on her own body. Believing that they are both free from infection and that they can both starve together, Mrs. Clennam accepts the marriage only to find out within a year that her husband has a mistress and a child—indeed, that he has known passion and pleasure. The sickness she feared most (sexual and psychological intimacy and contact) had already infected him.

In what she thinks will offer her protection, Mrs. Clennam terminates communication between the two lovers and raises the "lost boy" (Arthur) as her own in the hope (or "half-hop[e]") that he will love her (810, 824). Such a confinement, which she enforces to rewrite the narrative of her life with Arthur, fails. She felt the "consequences" of the sinners' love, and as she explains it to Rigaud, rather than bring her closer to Arthur's father it further isolated her from him: "Arthur's father and I lived no farther apart, with half the globe between us, than when we were together in this house" (810). Her initial desire that her husband would be someone with whom she could identify and connect was destroyed. Instead, she experienced the type of isolation that she would spend the rest of her life (save for one brief and rather gothic moment when she goes to Amy Dorrit) cultivating. Only through such isolation does she maintain—or believe she maintains—any affiliation with Arthur, as he is the only one who knows what it means to be raised with a "restraining and correcting hand." Mrs. Clennam becomes uncharacteristically desperate to preserve this one form of contact, no matter how limited it might be. If the story reaches Arthur, she will lose his respect and that "empty place in his heart," which not even he understands (824). She is wrong; or rather, the type of touch she advocates—one that is restraining and correcting—is wrong.

Unlike Miss Wade's attempt to transmit her story, Mrs. Clennam's is successful. That is, she finds someone who has the superior capacity—whose primary purpose in the novel is—to provide salubrious contact. In this way, Mrs. Clennam attempts to maintain her fragile bond to Arthur's story, thus evincing to the reader the ideal of quarantine. Mrs. Clennam incorporated Amy Dorrit into her isolation shortly before the novel's beginning. We learn of Amy Dorrit's presence in Mrs. Clennam's room during Arthur's first visit home. She is the only person to whom Mrs. Clennam ever reaches out, which we first see in an odd moment of contact that astonishes Affrey: when "Mrs. Clennam put out her hand, and laid it on [Amy's] arm" and then "she drew down her face and kissed her on the forehead" (364). Amy offers Mrs. Clennam protection, as she promises to absorb and safely dispose of Mrs. Clennam's secret, though not without "confid[ing] the general outline of [it] to Mr. Meagles" (839). To give the story to Amy, Mrs. Clennam must first "reclaim it" (822). She asks for the documents that Amy was supposed to give to Arthur and then returns the packet to Amy, asking her to read it and discover its contents. Mrs. Clennam takes back some of the control she had lost, and by physically handing the documents to Amy herself, she initiates the saving contact. Once Amy learns what has been done to her inheritance and to Arthur's heritage, she complies with Mrs. Clennam's command to preserve the link that binds them as mother and son: "Let me never feel, while I am still alive, that I die before his face, and utterly perish away from him, like one consumed by lightning and swallowed by an earthquake" (825). Mrs. Clennam requires only that she remain visible to Arthur, that she not "perish away" in some biblical catastrophe.

Touch is always revelatory and fortifying, and Amy Dorrit is its most dutiful practitioner. She functions—or tries to function—as a safe haven that, following the logic of quarantine, protects good but also keeps bad in and transforms it into good, into plot and narrative. Throughout the novel, when we turn our attention to Amy, we are repeatedly surprised that she is more Florence Dombey than Little Nell. Arthur, Flora, and the prostitute she meets on the street are all shocked that she can survive the cold. On the evening that Amy comes to Arthur's lodgings to thank him for his kindness, he "happen[s] to touch [her foot]" and comments that it is "like marble" (183). And later, she must assure her friends, "I am quite well" (301), as when she meets Pet at St. Bernard's Hospice. In this episode, the health of both women provides the means for bringing them together. After Pet, who is pregnant, faints, Amy nurses her but must preemptively assuage any concern over her own health. Pet invites Amy to stay by her bedside, though she fears it will be too cold, and Amy explains what we already know to be true from the night she was locked out of her "home": "I don't mind cold. I am not delicate, if I look so" (468).

The novel moves toward Amy's version of touch and quarantine, which, though it does not appear to be much, is a significant force. Amy is immune to suspicion, having grown up under a cloud of it all her life. Three brief moments of contact help to illustrate the range of Amy's reach. In the first, Amy's sister, Fanny, scolds her for being seen in public with Mr. Nandy, whose brand of poverty the Dorrits find unacceptable. Amy asks her simply, "Does it disgrace anybody . . . to take care of this poor old man?" After her sister answers in the affirmative and accuses Amy of knowing the answer, Fanny moves "to the other side of the way" to be "unmolested." Amy, as if to counter her sister's isolationism, tells Mr. Nandy,

"[G]ive me your arm again" (390). In a second scene of impropriety, one that hints at literal as well as metaphorical contagion, Amy clasps a prostitute's hand, telling her, "I am not afraid of you." The woman claims, "I never should have touched you, but I thought you were a child," and then "with a strange and wild cry, she went away" (191). In the third scene of contact, Pancks asks her to "show [him] the palm of [her] hand," and even though she thinks he might be "mad," she complies, "hold[ing] out her left hand with the thimble in it." He takes it, "touching it with his blunt forefinger" and "tracing out a line in her hand with his clumsy finger." We do not yet know what kind of character he is (good or bad), but through this contact, Pancks is revealed to be "a brighter and gentler-looking man than she [or we] supposed him to be" (307). In these scenes of contact, Amy gives Mr. Nandy her arm, the prostitute her hand, and Pancks her wrist; in what will become the most important connection of all, she gives Arthur her heart.

Her most significant act of contact, however, occurs when she attaches Mrs. Clennam's story to her own, recalling her childhood in the "poor prison" as a way of proving that even the most dire circumstances need not lead to "angry feelings and unforgiving deeds" (825). She urges Mrs. Clennam to "[b]e guided only by the healer of the sick, the raiser of the dead, the friend of all who were afflicted and forlorn, the patient Master who shed tears of compassion for our infirmities." Amy directs the language of health to one who has been raised from a form of death herself. It is advice we know that Amy has followed or attempts to follow herself; it is advice, however, that, when read through the lens of quarantine, wherein touch is both cultivated and also limited, provides hope.[61] Although Amy fixates her attention on her sick, afflicted, forlorn, and infirm father (almost to the exclusion of others), she does offer herself as a traveling cordon sanitaire for a dejected few, having been immunized by her "defective" upbringing against both filth and contagion (826).

Given the novel's interest in delimited touch, it should come as no surprise that it ends by bringing Amy and Arthur together in a final quarantine. For although Arthur is in the Marshalsea prison at the end of the novel, his sickness and subsequent care have more to do with contagion than with criminality. (Rigaud even refers to the Marshalsea as a hospital for imbeciles.) This is not to say that prison is a metaphor for quarantine but that in it, as in quarantine, touch defines and shapes the narrative encounters, reminding us of our physical (our somatic) connection to and responsibility for our own stories as well as the stories of those around us. Arthur's investments with Merdle (specifically, his investment of Doyce's money) precipitate his collapse, but Arthur's illness is strictly a family matter that began long ago. His parents get ill, go insane, become catatonic, and die. But while his imprisonment and illness begin familiarly enough—each of his parents suffers a medical response to isolation or exile—his trajectory takes on a much different cast. We know from the moment that John Chivery—who finds that he cannot shake hands with Arthur—gives him Mr. Dorrit's former room in the Marshalsea that Arthur's story will find connection. The room is a space that Arthur believes was "sanctified" by Amy; where once Arthur saw the "taint" of the "prison atmosphere" on Little Dorrit, now he imagines the overwhelming presence of Little Dorrit in the prison atmosphere and on the prison walls. This does not mean that the taint is gone; rather, its infectiousness creates a bond between Amy and Arthur. Alone in John's room, the room that used to be Amy's, Arthur becomes overwhelmed by the memory of her presence and "la[ys] his hands on the insensible wall, as tenderly as if it had been herself that he touched" (757). When John attempts to speak of Amy's love for Arthur, it becomes clear that Arthur does not fully comprehend, and John must not only name the man of her affection ("You!") but also must physically remind Arthur who that "You" is. He "touch[es] [Arthur] with the back of his hand up on the breast" (762). This connection with Amy through John's touch convinces Arthur to revise the narrative he constructed around his Little Dorrit. He rethinks the past with this new information in mind: the kiss he gave her the day her father was released from debtor's prison and she fainted, and the letters she wrote to him from abroad all have "new meaning" (764). A new plot emerges, which is to say, the one that was always already there.

Arthur's reaction to the "place," to the atmosphere, invokes a sanitary model of narrative, one designed to tidy things up and accelerate closure. But such a distinction between sanitation and quarantine would be misleading. Initially, the Marshalsea is too much for Arthur to bear, largely because it appears to isolate him from his Little Dorrit.[62] He imagines what a tragedy it would have been if they had acted on their love before his incarceration. The narrator explains, "Granted that she loved him, and he had known it and had suffered himself to love her, what a road to have led her away upon—the road that would have brought her back to this miserable place!" (766). His "dread and hatred of the place became so intense that he felt it a labor to draw his breath in it" (787). He develops a "slow fever" and eventually becomes insensible, losing track of people and time, as a result of his anxiety and sorrow. As if in answer to his "longing for other air[,] . . . some abiding impression of a garden st[eals] over him—a garden of flowers, with a damp warm wind gently stirring their scents" (789). The beauty and fragrance of the flowers that Little Dorrit leaves for Arthur revive his senses and his spirit. With Little Dorrit comes the fresh air Arthur so desperately needs. She comes to him in her old dress with an "old friend," Maggy, who helps to make the environment "fresh and neat" and provides necessary supplies for the invalid room. Sanitation and quarantine blur, as the lovers are connected and Arthur is cleansed, but it is not until Arthur's debt has been paid and Amy can prove her poverty that their plots and lives can unite. He asks her not to visit him "soon or often," because he believes that the prison is "now a tainted place, and . . . [that] the taint of it clings to [him]" (794). He imagines "brighter and better scenes" for Little Dorrit, forgetting that as the Child of the Marshalsea she is immune to its taint, having "[drunk] from infancy of a well whose waters had their own peculiar stain, their own unwholesome and unnatural taste" (86). Little Dorrit needs no cure. This contaminated well may have stunted her growth, but it replaces size with a kind of fortitude unprecedented in the novel.

The prison, then, gets redeemed not by sanitation but by a "stained" individual, whose ethereal touch goes almost unnoticed, certainly underappreciated, until the end of the novel. The beginning of the final chapter reinforces the irony of quarantine as a unifying device and as a place of health. The narrator begins, "On a healthy autumn day, the Marshalsea prisoner, weak but otherwise restored, sat listening to a voice that read to him" (847). The passage aligns healthy autumn with Amy, the contaminated former (or perpetual) prisoner; we are asked to focus our attention not on the atmosphere but on a voice, a *person.* It is a scene best imagined as quarantine, for Arthur and Amy are brought together not to be cured but to be isolated—"inseparable and blessed"—from the world around them. If anything, we might object to their sequestration and to the way Dickens excludes other forms of contact in the end. For while the narrator tells us that Amy's brother and sister will share their part in her life, "the noisy and the eager, and the arrogant and the froward and the vain" will not. This is the story that quarantine allows Dickens to tell, one that imagines connection framed by isolation, one that imagines hope as a form of prevention. We can see in their union how persons and touch, the things that define quarantine, become, for the reformer who believes quarantine is mistaken, a way for the novelist to connect plots, unite characters, and tell a healthy tale.

Chapter Four

The Omniscience of Invalidism

The Case of Harriet Martineau

Despite, or perhaps because of, the Victorian preoccupation with health, one of the most idealized figures in the literature and culture of the period was not the robust, sociable hero but the delicate, isolated invalid. Although these invalids are not generally the Victorian novel's primary character, they often function as a powerful center around which the narrative's action develops and around which stories about health unfold. From Jane Austen's feeble though strategic Mrs. Smith to Charlotte Yonge's wise, wheelchair-bound Ermine Williams and George Eliot's vengeful, bedridden valetudinarian Peter Featherstone, the chronically ill were everywhere in the novel, interfering with and enhancing the stories of their conventionally healthy counterparts. And by century's end, readers were sick of them.

The invalids who were particularly annoying were not the complainers and curmudgeons but the ones who became almost divine as a result of their condition. As the writer of "An Invalid's Grievance" (1887) claims, open up a novel and "you are gravely assured that beauty, talent, goods, nay every gift desired by man, varies in inverse proportion to health. [The novelist's] heroines—for I must confess this species of fetishism is generally reserved for ladies, though from time to time, men come in for their share—become more and more beautiful, amiable, and unselfish as their strength fades away. The little frailties inherent in them as human beings gradually disappear; their minds, no matter how dull in the days of their strength, in weakness become transcendent in penetration and judgment."[1] "The cruelest rub of all," he continues, has less to do with their talent and beauty than with the supposed intellectual improvement that comes from sustained illness. The writer sneers, "No doubt a whole day spent wondering whether that confounded pain will ever cease its gnawing will have a marvelous effect in brightening my intellect and rendering my penetration more acute, my arguments more convincing" (443). Even those who achieve "transcendent virtues" (443) as a result of their state must experience a loss of reality, of innate humanness: "They [that is, nonfictional invalids] are no longer men and brethren, but something beyond—above if you will—the ken of poor weak mortals" (444). This writer fixates on a particular version of invalidism, one that saw a transcendent vitality in disability, arguing that all would be well—or at least, the sick could simply be sick in peace—if novelists would only adhere to the "beauty of realism" instead of promoting a "fanciful" and "unnatural" ideal about illness (443). For this aggrieved invalid, the fictional ones are simply too much of the wrong kind of fiction.

The invalids featured in popular novels, as this writer laments, do not represent sickness as it really is; their conditions essentially mark them not as the opposite of health but as a version of health, reappropriating it for a larger purpose. Maria Frawley argues in *Invalidism and Identity in Nineteenth-Century Britain* that the "term" *invalid* was flexible, "serv[ing] a wide range of purposes" and referring to a variety of social and medical roles.[2] Frawley's work focuses primarily on the range of "sick roles" that invalids construct and inhabit, but she notes that "'[i]nvalid' is also related etymologically to 'invalescence,' defined in one instance as 'the state of condition of being an invalid, ill health,' yet in another as 'to be strong against' and 'strength; health; force.'"[3] As in the plots of prevention we see from Austen in chapter 1, the invalid's value—though it would seem to come from a failure of prevention—centers, I argue here, precisely on her role as an agent of it: the invalid is simultaneously a cautionary tale, the teller of healthy tales, and a narrative of "strength; health; force." Invalidism, like prevention, produces highly developed foresight, the ability to project, to fantasize, and to narrate. The invalid, particularly one who suffers from a chronic, incurable condition, may sit on the sidelines ready to watch, report, and guide, but she is no wretch in need of cure. Such invalids represent a desire for maintenance and a resistance to the traditional cure narrative that, as I argue in previous chapters, defines health. This is not simply a theoretical desire, for although the invalid's claims to health may seem dubious to us "weak mortals," it is through the novel and through omniscience that her health becomes legible, reaffirming the medical views about health's capaciousness I discuss in chapter 2.

Invalids, whether they come from fiction or nonfiction, do not generally function as models of health or of narration.[4] Indeed, as I suggest earlier, Jane Eyre's narrative identity requires physical wellness. Invalids tend to be seen in terms of their cultural, political, and aesthetic value. There are those dying darlings—such as Helen Burns, Little Eva, and Paul Dombey—who are too good for the vanities of this mortal world. Their conditions make us weep, repent, and reform. Then there are those who tend toward the cranky, the demanding, and the just plain odd. Mr. Woodhouse fixates on himself, oblivious to everything but his own alimental remedies; Linton Heathcliff is a sniveling pawn in his father's revenge tragedy; Mr. Fairlie's selfishness marks him as morally suspect and socially dangerous. These are hardly model citizens worth emulating, and they are certainly not worth listening to. Such characters—even the ethereal Paul—lack the permanence and stability to function as a narrator does, as the omniscient narrator must.

The "transcendent invalid" is the one who interests me, and the one who best expands our understanding of health. And although they were annoying to some, such invalids were a popular character type throughout the first half of the nineteenth century. Their "peculiar privilege,"[5] as Harriet Martineau would call it, came to be invested with a form of knowledge that was deemed morally superior and socially necessary. In 1866, an essay in the *Saturday Review* focuses on the importance of such invalids, lamenting that the "angelic being with a weak spine, who, from her sofa, directed with mild wisdom the affairs of the family or the parish" has been replaced by bigamists and murders.[6] This argument, which lauds the works of "pre-Braddonian" lady novelists such as Craik and Yonge, is as much about the novel's form as about the characters it produces, focusing, like the "Invalid's Grievance," on the novel-as-culprit and tacitly acknowledging the genre's role in shaping perception and instructing people (for good and for ill) on how to act and what to do. While such a view of fiction's power is not unique to narratives featuring invalids, the connection these writers draw between novels and physical debility locates the figure of the invalid—her way of knowing and her role in the story and in society—within a framework of novelistic invention and fantasy. Such a critique invites us to consider not only what novels do to invalids (as the "Invalid's Grievance" does) but also what invalids do to, and for, the novel. This influence works both ways: invalids turn to novelists when justifying their social relevance, and novelists turn to the invalid when finding a socially relevant way to narrate the plots of their fictional ones. Regardless of whether they are beloved, these "angels" provide novelists with more than a few cloying or beneficent minor characters; conversely, the novel offers the invalid more than a guide to becoming an idealized version of herself.

Not only does novelistic fiction of the period absorb the qualities of invalidism that were developed by Martineau and others but also the figure of the invalid draws on the omniscience perfected by novelists to imagine and justify her unique social position and make a claim for her healthier perspective. As stable observers with no (or very minimal) plots of their own, narrators and invalids share the capacity and desire to observe and direct the plots of those around them. And while significant differences exist between the two conditions—for example, when suffering from chronic debility one is not generally referred to as "omniscient"—both states rely on transcending the material conditions of the physical body to create the kind of privileged and distanced knowledge that has the capacity to make order out of chaos and the power to see enough, know all, and tell the stories of others.

As a writer who is decidedly more famous for her views on political economy and her invalidism than for her novels, Harriet Martineau offers a unique vantage point from which to study this affiliation between invalids and narrators. She is outside of the canon of the Victorian novel but also invested in its success and committed to its aims. As such, she exemplifies the social and fictional relationship between the two roles, demonstrating what it means to inhabit both positions. Her novel *Deerbrook* (1839) and her memoir *Life in the Sick-Room* (1844) register her personal stake in asserting the "peculiar privileges" of narrators and invalids by depicting the interdependence of the two conditions. Taken together, her works perform the reciprocity between novels and invalids that I am suggesting underwrites the emergent cultural authority of both.

In many ways, these narratives allowed Martineau to invent a character in fiction and in her personal life that later novelists would turn to when narrating their own fictions. Charles Dickens's *Master Humphrey's Clock* (1840–41) invokes but then abandons the invalid narrator; Emily Brontë's *Wuthering Heights* (1847) uses Lockwood's temporary incapacity as an occasion for narration; Phineas Fletcher in Dinah Mulock Craik's popular *John Halifax, Gentleman* (1856) struggles to reconcile his duty as first-person narrator of John's story with his personal need to be the healthy hero or to keep the healthy hero to himself; Elizabeth Gaskell uses the invalid's sofa to frame and organize her collection of short stories in *Round the Sofa*

(1859).[7] These "narrators," though central to the production of their respective stories, do not achieve the level or degree of omniscience and health that Martineau imagined for herself and her characters. Craik's narrator comes closest to fulfilling Martineau's vision; but by dividing Phineas between his roles as a desiring character, on the one hand, and as a reliable, even omniscient narrator, on the other, Craik allows the hero's story to become one overtly about the narrator and the possibility of healthy narration.

For Martineau, as the following pages demonstrate, this tension between duty and desire never overwhelms the invalid, as her capacity for omniscience and her place in the narrative remain fixed and provide the ordering perspective that Jonathan Arac claims for the novelist. In *Commissioned Spirits,* Arac explains, "The chaos of the urban experience fostered a wish for a clarifying overview," and the novelist "arrogated the power of 'commissioned spirits' [articulated by Wordsworth in the *Prelude*] to set their readers, along with themselves, in a position of overview, as if pinnacled high above the world they viewed."[8] The novelist, as I have been suggesting, was not the only one to fill this role. The "transcendent invalid" was equally invested in claiming this "overview" position, imbuing her "special" and "peculiar" perspective with a form of knowledge that, for a time, the culture needed. As Frawley explains, invalidism is as much a "cultural mentality [and] a mode of thought" as it is a mark of one's identity.[9] This "mentality" and the purpose to which it was ostensibly put are valuable to the novelist whose narrators explicitly and implicitly claim this perspective. And invalidism, like omniscience, emerges as a particular—"peculiar"—way of seeing and of knowing the world and determining "what health is."

Martineau was not, of course, the first to assert the invalid's privilege. In 1827, the *Christian Spectator* devoted an essay to the so-called privileges of invalids, observing, "The situation of the invalid, with the concomitant appendages of pain and sickness, the pill and bitter draught, solitary days and 'wearisome nights,' the restrictions necessarily imposed, and the privations to which he is subject, has very little to excite the envy of the world, which 'places its bliss in action,' or luxurious 'ease,' in parade, and noise, and bustle, and (may I not add?) in vanity. But the world knows little of what may be enjoyed, even under all those seeming disadvantages."[10]

Invalids do not see the world as others do; their vision, which is shaped by pain and solitude, becomes more acute, and as a result the invalid is "rendered more extensively useful to mankind, than if blessed with health to participate in the active duties of life."[11] Removed from the bustle and parade, these invalids, at least according to this essayist, are outsiders looking on with clarity and purpose; physical limitations free the mind to contemplate the many truths of the self, humanity, and the world. Rather than complain incessantly or die gloriously, this class of invalids sits on the sidelines to observe, think, and act for a greater good.

Edward Bulwer Lytton articulates a similar view of the mind's narrativizing powers in an essay in *The Student,* which Martineau read before penning her memoir on invalidism:[12] "Every one of us must have observed that during a lengthened illness the mind acquires the habit of making to itself a thousand sources of interest . . . out of that quiet monotony which seems so unvaried to ordinary eyes. We grow usually far more susceptible to commonplace impressions:—As one whose eyes are touched by a fairy spell, a new world opens to us out of the surface of the tritest things."[13] For Bulwer and others, the enforced stillness and isolation of the body during illness imbue "ordinary" vision and knowledge with the ability to create a new world—a narrative—out of the everyday. The same qualities touted as unique to the invalid—the ability to see something special in the everyday—are among the qualities that characterize the novel's authoritative perspective and its rise as the period's dominant genre. The stasis associated with invalidism affords a mobility of mind that resonates with omniscient narrators of the traditional novel.

The critical discussion surrounding narrative point of view offers various ways to understand this affiliation.[14] Particularly relevant is the way we imagine the narrator's presence in fiction, and how the insight gained from this position transforms into a duty. Audrey Jaffe offers a generous definition of omniscience that applies to the invalid's narrative powers. In *Vanishing Points,* Jaffe argues, "What we call omniscience can be located . . . not in presence or absence, but in the tension between the two." As she describes it, "[O]mniscience in general . . . is a fantasy: of unlimited knowledge and mobility; of transcending the boundaries imposed by the physical being and by an ideology of unitary identity."[15] This reading of omniscience, though specifically referring to Dickens's novels, speaks as well to the ways that invalids write about themselves and their condition—and also how a particular class of invalids functions in the Victorian novel.[16] While the invalid characters I discuss here are also characters in the story, the cultural understanding (and narrative construction) of the invalid's power marks their presence in the narrative as a form of absence, their knowledge as a form of transcendence, their being as "beyond the ken."

More than simply *being* omniscient (like a narrator), the invalid becomes a sign of or synonym for omniscience. To be sure, significant differences exist between the two conditions—when confined to bed with chronic illness, for example, one is not referred to as "an omniscient," and severe pain obscures rather than heightens vision. Yet both states of being (invalidism and omniscience) rely to some degree on existing outside of the material condition of the physical body to create the kind of privileged and distanced and thus healthy knowledge that, as we see in Martineau's works, energizes plots and engages readers.

Believing that recovery was unlikely, Martineau wrote *Life in the Sick-Room* during a five-year confinement for an ovarian tumor, which resulted in the prolapse of her uterus. Covering a range of topics from pain and endurance to homeopathy and mesmerism to the penny post and privacy, *Life in the Sick-Room* stands out among sickroom literature of the period because of its emphasis on the invalid's mental capacity and agency.[17] As Frawley notes, "Sickness was not only the linchpin of [Martineau's] self-understanding, her guiding frame of reference, it was the lens through which she wanted her readers to see and understand her life and career."[18] But such "sickness," as I have been suggesting, gets transformed, particularly in Martineau's novel *Deerbrook,* by its affinity with omniscience; sickness is not health's opposite. Or, rather, it is not only that.

Like "An Invalid's Grievance" and Bulwer Lytton's *The Student,* Martineau's writings continually assert that the invalid's removal constitutes a privilege rather than a dilemma, a healthy stance rather than a sick one. They demonstrate the tension between invalidism as a social and medical problem to be cured and invalidism as a necessary condition of social duty and narrative action to be preserved. Martineau goes further than the writers of these earlier works to articulate a model for invalid behavior that relies heavily on literary principles, particularly on a principle of omniscience. In *Life in the Sick-Room,* she explains to her fellow invalids, "By our being withdrawn from the disturbing bustles of life in the world; by our leisure for reading and contemplation of various sides of questions, and by our singular opportunities for quiet reflection, we must, almost necessarily, see further than we used to do, and further than many others do on subjects of interest, which involve general principles" (116–17). The narrated (rather than the lived) version of the invalid experience is not so much about diagnosis, treatment, and the desired cure; it is about seeing the "old" in a "new," truer, way.[19] In an effort to express fully what this position is like and how it works, Martineau finds an analogy in poetry. She likens the invalid's powers to the seraphs she read about as a child in the works of John Milton and Mark Akenside, "poised on balanced wing, watching the bringing out a world from chaos" (78). The young Martineau "longed for the privilege of the supposed seraph," and the invalid Martineau believed she had found it: "Though I, and my fellow in lot, must wait long for the seraphic powers, which would enable us fully to enjoy and use our position, we have the position" (78). This "position" so assertively demanded for the invalid by Martineau becomes an important marker of omniscience in Victorian fiction.

The seraphic figure Martineau uses to describe the invalid's role is strikingly similar to the imagery used by nineteenth-century novelists to describe narrative perspective and novelistic authority. The "good spirit" in Dickens's *Dombey and Son* (1848) and the "shadow" of semiomniscience he imagined as directing *Household Words* share common ground with the invalid who, although immobile, has the same theoretical ability to lift the rooftops off of the city's houses to reveal the action inside.[20] The invalid sits apart from society to gain a perspective that enables him or her to see and have knowledge about the larger picture of the world.[21] Omniscience, therefore, does not simply describe the actual form of narration—*Life in the Sick-Room* is, after all, narrated in the first person. Rather, it describes a way of knowing and of being that is central to the novel and to Victorian conceptions of the invalid's identity.

While Martineau theorizes fully the power of the seraph-like perspective in *Life in the Sick-Room,* her novel *Deerbrook* (1839) first demonstrates how this kind of privilege is central to her authority as a novelist. It is here—in the novel, not the memoir—that Martineau essentially invents the invalid. The popularity of *Life in the Sick-Room* and subsequent controversy about Martineau's cure continues to overshadow *Deerbrook*'s importance to understanding Martineau's invalidism.[22] Written five years before the memoir, the novel shaped how Martineau imagined the invalid's—and thus the narrator's—privileged perspective. Generally considered an early example of domestic realism—as one of the few transitional novels to bridge the gap between Jane Austen and the Brontës—*Deerbrook* does not at first appear to concern itself with invalidism. Told from a third-person omniscient perspective, *Deerbrook* follows the love plots of Margaret and Hester Ibbotson. The sisters, aged twenty and twenty-one, respectively, have just moved from Birmingham after the death of their father and are ideal candidates for the marriage market. Their Aunt Grey wastes no time in speculating about Hester's prospects with the eligible apothecary, Mr. Hope. The kind, intelligent doctor falls in love with Margaret, only to realize that everyone else, including both sisters, believes he has been courting the prettier but intellectually inferior sister, Hester. Bound by a sense of duty, Hope marries Hester, and the three live together until the end of the novel, when, after overcoming numerous obstacles, Margaret marries the town's other eligible bachelor, Philip Enderby.

The main action of *Deerbrook*,[23] therefore, comes from the crisis and recovery that mark the marriage plots of Hester and Hope and Margaret and Enderby, but it is through a fifth character, the crippled governess, Maria Young, that Martineau anchors the novel's narrative point of view and not only disrupts the closural value of metaphorical health but also transforms the very meaning of health. Before the novel's beginning, Maria was on her way to becoming the heroine of her own domestic tale. The narrator tells us that "there had been some gossip . . . that Philip Enderby would be Maria's lover, when he should be old enough to think of marrying" (48). In fact, Philip Enderby admits to Margaret that "some [of his] boyish dreams connected themselves to Maria Young" (338). This plot never developed, however, because a gig accident that killed her father (her only living relative) "lamed [her] for life" (48). As a result, Maria deemed herself "out of the game" (46) and became a governess for the two main families of Deerbrook—the Greys and the Rowlands (Philip Enderby's sister). Removed from one important narrative role, she relocated to a position of philosophical and moral overview, representing and narrating ideal health.[24] No mere fifth wheel, Maria demonstrates what happens when the marriage plot fails and the invalid lives on, when the recovery from a crisis does not always lead to closure.[25]

Certainly, this novel could be told without Maria Young—indeed, as scholars are fond of pointing out, a version of *Deerbrook* was told better by George Eliot in *Middlemarch*. But this story is *not* told without her; in fact, Maria becomes central to its telling. Critics describe Maria as the most "complex" and "absorbing" character of the whole novel, but because she is often "used to articulate feminist ideas," most scholars focus their analysis on the politics of her role as single woman and governess.[26] To substantiate this interpretation, they are drawn to a scene toward the novel's end in which Margaret asks Maria about employment opportunities for women. Maria tells Margaret about the few options available to educated women; she can be a teacher, an artist, or a writer, although the latter two should not "be regarded as resources for bread" (515). Moments such as these led the critic Valerie Sanders to claim, "*Deerbrook* may be read as an exploration of the narrow futures available for single women of reduced means, strong sensibilities, and no very tempting exterior."[27] The governess/single-woman matrix seems to animate Maria's role in the novel—in this capacity, she grounds the novel in real-world concerns about the very limited opportunities women such as Martineau had for supporting themselves. If, however, this were Maria's primary role, why must she be "crippled"? In part, Maria's invalidism keeps her from invading the marriage plot, as later literary governesses do. More important, while her status registers the cultural attitude (and novelistic fetish) that often conflated women with invalids, Maria offers an alternative narrative through which to reconsider how both invalids and narrators function as a presence that is also a necessary absence.

Martineau took a personal interest in this question when she went to write *Life in the Sick-Room*. Critics rarely discuss the parallels between *Deerbrook* and *Life in the Sick-Room*. Sanders hints at a link between the two texts when she notes, in passing, that Martineau's use of the seraph in *Life in the Sick-Room* "was, perhaps, just a logical extension of Maria Young's position in *Deerbrook*."[28] Instead of exploring the ways in which the rhetoric and imagery Martineau uses in *Life in the Sick-Room* were developed in her depiction of Maria Young in *Deerbrook*, critics generally focus on the notion that Maria is *like* Martineau, "a kind of alter-ego figure."[29] In some ways, however, the reverse is true—Martineau became like

Maria Young, for writing this character taught her how to speak as both an invalid and a narrator. While certain elements of Maria's story can and should be read in terms of the "cult of feminine invalidism," we must also recognize the ways in which Martineau removes the invalid (male or female) from the social realm—from the invalid couch—and repositions her in relation to the novel's form, particularly its narration. In this sense, the invalid ceases to function as a historical figure and becomes more a figure of omniscience, of the ways that stories get told. Her body, emptied of its biological potential, gets written into the structure of the story and becomes an agent of knowledge, a technique of narrative overview.

Martineau introduces Maria and the key elements that link chronic invalidism to narration early in the novel, and these are, at first, physical and spatial rather than wholly spiritual or mental. During the Ibbotsons' first visit to Maria at her schoolroom, Hester asks Maria whether she "spend[s] all of [her] time here." Maria offers a very forthcoming explanation: "Almost the whole day. I have a lodging in the village; but I leave it early these fine mornings, and stay here till dark. I am so lame as to make it inconvenient to pass over the ground oftener than necessary; and I find it pleasanter to see trees and grass through every window here, than to look out into the farrier's yard,—the only prospect from my lodging" (28). For Maria, questions about how she uses her time entail descriptions of her body. She spends most of the day at the schoolhouse, because her physical condition makes it difficult to go anywhere else. But rather than dwell on the "inconveniences" of her lameness, she immediately links her debility to the act of looking from her lodgings and from her workplace—in fact, she derives a knowing pleasure from it. This early correspondence between Maria's "lameness" and vision establishes her function as a stationary observer who, as we will see, often guides the narrative experience in a way that noninvalids, at least within Martineau's novel, cannot.

Maria's introduction not only invokes a connection between immobility and heightened perspective but also indicates the role that solitude plays in the development of the invalid's narrative powers. When Maria continues her description of the difference between the view from her lodgings and the view from the schoolroom, she explains, "The furnace and sparks are pretty enough on a winter's evening, especially when one is too ill or dismal to do anything but watch them; but at this season one grows so tired of old horse-shoes and cinders; and so I sit here" (28). By ending with "and so I sit here," Maria confirms her isolation, which allows us to imagine her perched at her window as a static observer and prepares us for her role as a locus of narration and an authority that presides like the good spirit over the events of the plot. Margaret and Hester, and perhaps the reader, sense "a world of desolation in these words" (28), but as we learn during one of Maria's solitary musings later in the novel, she will not be pitied. For Maria, "to be alone, and to be let alone, . . . is to be put in the post of observation on others" (46–47). Martineau makes a distinction here between being "alone" and being "let alone"; solitude means being alone, but it also means being free from the demands that come with marriage and family.[30]

Her alternative position does not, however, come without its own duties. That is, being a woman who is "not to have . . . a home [and] an intimate" means having the responsibility to act on behalf of others. Maria tells herself and the reader that "[w]ithout daring to meddle, one may stand clear-sighted, ready to help" (44). Even as it reflects an aspect of domesticity that figures women solely as helpmates, this passage points to an alternative form of action for the invalid, one that registers an ethics inherent to observation and storytelling. Maria is not content simply to observe and record; she has responsibilities attached to this vision. For Maria, this kind of "seeing" demands a keen imagination, which she says is "a better medium than the eye" (45). Maria assumes that she has the ability and, in fact, the authority to watch and to guide others. Her physical condition, more than her gender, here, helps to establish Maria's power to "stand clear-sighted."[31] Such counsel has a decidedly novelistic quality. To be sure, Maria is by vocation a teacher and confidante, continually modeling practical advice and admonishing immoral behavior, but her place in the novel is initially defined in literary terms. She is, above all, a storyteller, a narrator.

We first witness Maria in this role when she sits at her window during an unexpected holiday from work. Her internal monologue at the window defines her as a peripheral figure while demonstrating the dynamism of her stasis: "'It is a luxury,' thought the gazer, 'for one who cannot move about to sit here and look abroad. I wonder whether I should have been with the party if I had not been lame'" (44). Her initial tentativeness (her position is at first a luxury and then an obstacle) signals a remnant of desire left over from her initial romance plot. And although Maria could "move about" if necessary and with assistance, as we see later in the novel when Mr. Hope provides her a pony, she chooses to remain indoors, sitting at her window, contemplating the "party" before her. This choice highlights the invalid's relationship to narrative time: retrospection and projection, as old plots versus new plots all come under her purview. By referring to Maria as "the gazer," a term Martineau used later to describe the invalid in *Life in the Sick-Room*, the narrator emphasizes the degree to which stasis and observation signify agency and narrative privilege.[32] She is not labeled in terms of her social role as "the governess" or her physical status as "the invalid" or "cripple" at this point. Rather, she is represented by her actions, as one who sees and knows and tells; her disabled body limits mobility and as a result fades into the background, as her mind and vision travel "about" and "abroad," and she takes comfort in pleasures of her condition.

Taking a cue from the Romantics, Maria explains her condition in relation to memory ("the mind's eye") and narrative. People like herself, she notes, find "pleasure . . . more in the recollection of . . . natural enjoyments than at the moment" (45) of experience, particularly when they "see others tripping over commons and through fields where [they] cannot go" (46). Maria explains the benefits of imagination, musing that Byron could not write about Lake Leman until he was "within four walls" and that the opening lines of *Paradise Lost* far surpass any sunrises she has personally experienced.[33] Maria convinces herself that "[o]nce having received pictures into our mind's eye, and a clear eye in the mind to see them with, the going about and obtaining more is not of very great consequence" (45). This detour into Maria's thoughts is a curious one. Instead of using Maria simply to comment on what her students or the main characters are doing in the novel, Martineau uses her to remove us from the immediate action and to express a philosophy of perspective and overview.[34]

But within this philosophy, we sense a slight tug between the enjoyment of participation and the enjoyment of imagination and observation. As Maria reminds us, the imagination we use when reading poetry or "good descriptions in books" (45) far surpasses any enjoyment we might experience from physical mobility. A good narrator makes us long to read; he keeps us invested in the text and glad we are there. Maria constructs her identity within this framework, for although she does not articulate a precise analogue (she is not like Byron, who gets to experience and then recall and write), Maria does draw on her memories. She creates in the moment, as she sits within the four walls. By attaching Maria's body and philosophy to the experience of reading, Martineau recasts the invalid as representing narrative potential rather than the narrative ends that her medical condition implies. And while she does not transfer this narrative authority completely to Maria, Martineau does construct this character in terms of omniscience.

Maria's impulse to tell stories and her "semiomniscience" become more overt when she describes and speculates to herself about what she sees but cannot hear: "O, there are the children! So that is their cowslip meadow! How like children they all look together, down on the grass!—gathering cowslips, I suppose. The two in black are more eager about it than Sophia. She sits on the stile while they are busy. The children are holding forth to their cousins—teaching them something, evidently" (46). She creates a vignette that works within a preestablished fictional structure, as she assumes the impending love story and projects the eventual pain. While her description sets the scene for the reader, Maria is limited in what she can offer in this role as "substitute narrator."[35] She can only "suppose" they are gathering cowslips and speculate that the children are "teaching something." Maria's limitations at this moment could be represented by any character caught on the other side of the glass, but Martineau locates this experience only in Maria, and in so doing represents the possibility of being outside of the action of the plot yet central to its narration.[36] Although it would have been possible for Maria to become "part of the party" if she had asked, she remains fixed inside to speculate and to enjoy her privacy, as if to protect her privilege as spectator and her relationship to the reader. She moves from speculation about what the children are doing to imagining potential love plots for Margaret and Hester, noting, "The tempest of passion may be brewing under the soft sun," and hinting at two possible (traditional) conclusions: they will either be lucky in love or suffer from it (46). Martineau narrates through the invalid, using her to foreshadow the complications and detours that accompany any marriage plot. This sense of projection, which Jaffe identifies with narrative authority, marks Maria as more than an observant character within the diegesis. Certainly, other characters in the novel watch and gossip about imagined relationships and love plots, but the fact that Maria engages in this activity in solitude (for only the reader to hear) separates these two versions of speculation.[37]

This scene allows Maria increasing self-consciousness and narrative awareness; she intrudes on her own narrative, commenting at one point on her role as observer and would-be narrator. "I love to overlook people," she says, "—to watch them acting unconsciously, and speculate for them! It is the most tempting thing in the world to contrast the little affairs one sees them busy about, with the very serious ones that await them—that await every one" (46). Maria guides the narrative here by imagining or predicting the futures—the stories—that await the subjects of her gaze, in the process offering commentary on the way *Deerbrook*'s plot moves (or will move) from small affairs to big ones. Innocent matchmaking and neighborly feuds give way to more-serious events: broken engagements that ultimately result in happy marriages, death from fever, and repentance for lying. Although Maria does not reveal the substance of her speculations, she does presume to know that her subjects act "unconsciously," that they are unaware of their futures, in a way that narrators treat their characters.

The window frames the character's desire and capacity for narration, which come from physical transcendence. Like the rooftops for Dickens's good spirit, the window becomes the portal through which the invalid accesses private truths. For Martineau in *Life in the Sick-Room,* the window is so important that she must describe the ideal configuration for cultivating what Frawley calls "the omniscience of sick vision," and what I am arguing aligns invalidism and health.[38] Martineau explains in *Life in the Sick-Room* that "[w]e [invalids] should have the widest expanse of sky, for night scenery. We should have a wide expanse of land or water, for the sake of a sense of liberty" (67). Of course, "there must not be too much sea" (67), as such a view might become too hard on one's nerves. She goes on to describe the view from her window, which includes, among other things, a priory, grazing cows, a harbor "where there are frequent wrecks," children playing, lovers talking, maids working, and a farmer gossiping (68–69). Martineau periodically aids her view by the use of a telescope, simultaneously extending and narrowing her perspective. This shift between the panoramic and the telescopic demonstrates how the invalid, moving easily between the general and the specific or the community and the individual, takes on the qualities of a narrator of fiction. *Deerbrook*'s narrator moves frequently between general commentary and the thoughts and actions of a particular character.[39]

Life in the Sick-Room requires the centrality of the invalid's voice and a more conventional (at least initially) version of the illness/health divide in a way that *Deerbrook* does not. The memoir, after all, is by, about, and mostly for invalids. But the rhetorical similarities between the novel and the sickroom narrative speak to Martineau's dependence on the fictional invalid; for, like Maria Young, the narrator in this "story" (known only as "An Invalid") finds value in solitude and duty in observation. Martineau turns to the window as a key symbol of the invalid's narrative potency. Borrowing the content and, in particular, the window imagery from *Deerbrook,* Martineau explains in *Life in the Sick-Room,* "When I think of what I have seen with my own eyes from one back window, in the few years of my illness; of how indescribably clear to me are many truths of life from my observations of the doings of tenants of a single row of houses; it seems scarcely necessary to see more than the smallest sample, in order to analyze life in its entireness" (68–69). This passage positions the invalid as sociologist, as one who has the right and duty to speculate about and speak for large segments of society based on a random sampling.[40] But her description of her actions also undercuts this scientific sense by suggesting that something magical occurs when the invalid sits at her window—the truths of life are revealed without too much effort on the part of the observer. The tenants Martineau observes offer a "truth"—they have a story to tell—but we never hear the entire story. In fact, she boasts that although she could "fill a volume—an interesting one too—with a simple detail of what [she] ha[s] witnessed [,] . . . [she] must tell nothing" (89). Martineau only hints at some of these details she might include in this "volume," as she "look[s] forward to the time when the bad training of children—the petulancies of neighbours—the errors of the ménage—the irksome superstitions, and the seductions of intemperance, shall all have been annihilated by the spread of intelligence" (89). As the invalid-narrator in *Life in the Sick-Room* draws on her special vision to bring the reader into her perspective, she remains vague about the knowledge it reveals but clear that she guards that knowledge. The story becomes less important than the fact that the invalid has the ability to "see" it in its entirety.

When read in isolation, Martineau's invalid memoir offers a justification for the invalid's social relevance. When read in tandem with *Deerbrook* as part of a larger theory of invalidism, however, the memoir begins to look more like a portrait of the invalid's narratological function. The author of the "Invalid's Grievance" might argue that what we are seeing in *Life in the Sick-Room* is how masterfully the novel influences behavior—Martineau models her own invalidism after the fetishized "cripple" she created in her novel. But it is more than that, for we see in Maria and the anonymous invalid who narrates *Life in the Sick-Room* how narrative point of view gets constructed around the invalid's place in the world and in the plot.

This formal expression occurs in *Deerbrook* as Maria looks out her window at the cowslip party. After she asserts her love for "overlook[ing] people," Maria goes on to narrate a scene *before* the novel's narrator does. Maria notices "[h]ow the children are flying over the meadow toward that gentleman who is fastening his horse to the gate! Mr. Hope no doubt" (47). Five pages later, after the narrator tells us about Maria's past and moves on to some of the village gossip about Mr. Hope, we learn (from the narrator this time) that "Mr. Hope threw himself from his horse at the entrance of the meadow, fastened his steed to the gate, and joined the party. The children ran to him" (52). Maria and the narrator both use the word *fasten,* which joins these two scenes together and fixes this moment from the invalid's perspective. This repetition not only momentarily collapses the distinction between narrator and invalid but also allows Maria to be present in a scene even when she is not part of it and to see without being seen. Maria sees things and in ways others cannot because they are too busy participating in the bustle of the world and the plots of novels. Even when she is absent, she has a presence that helps move the story forward. In the reverse angle of the above scene, taken from the narrator's point of view, Maria is not mentioned—that is, nobody (not even the narrator) notices her sitting at the window, and she becomes a shadowy presence in the reader's memory. We forget even that she has been watching until the party meets up with Philip Enderby and they begin talking about her. Despite the limitations on Maria's omniscience in this moment, we get a sense that she is not completely in the dark about the contents of this interaction. Margaret explains to Philip that she and Maria met before breakfast and plan to study German together and goes on to observe that "if [Maria] were a man, she would be called philosophical" (62). This comment leads to a group discussion about Maria's social and physical status and an extended conversation about exactly what it means to be philosophical. Philip Enderby suggests, "It is a happy thing that she is philosophical in her circumstances, poor thing" (62). Maria is socially peripheral but narratively central, becoming a topic of conversation and a device that brings the two main characters, Margaret and Philip, together.

Even when she is decidedly "with the party," Maria still functions as an outsider, as if perpetually looking through her schoolroom window. During the children's tea party, which is held in the schoolhouse, the narrator directs our reading of the other characters through Maria. As the festivities get under way, the narrator notes, "Maria's pleasure was, as usual, in observing all that went on" (104). This vantage point provides the reader with a survey of the events: "[Maria] could see Mr. Hope's look of delight" with Margaret; "[s]he saw how he helped Mary pour out the tea"; "[s]he observed Mr. Rowland's somewhat stiff politeness to Hester"; "[s]he could see Mrs. Grey watching every strawberry and sugar plum that went down the throats of the little Rowlands"; "she saw Hester's color and manner change as Mr. Hope came and went" (104–5). She notices all of these details, we are told, while others speak to her about her superior "management" and offer her some of the treats. Any conversation she may be having is subordinate to her observations and her ability to direct our field of vision and reading experience.

This is not to say that Maria is the only silent observer in the novel. Morris (Hester and Margaret's maid and former nurse) demonstrates her ability to observe her beloved Hester's marital woes. Some characters, particularly Margaret, even notice when Maria seems out of sorts. At one point, the narrator describes Maria through Margaret's eyes. During a debate with Philip Enderby about the "art of wooing," Margaret "chanced to perceive that Maria's hand shook so that she could not guide her needle" (77). Although the reader knows about Maria's thwarted marriage plot, Margaret does not, and it does not occur to her to speculate, as Maria might in such a case, about a failed love plot involving the invalid. Maria sublimates any leftover feelings about marriage in the development of her philosophy and moves outside of the realm of lovelorn governess.[41] This remnant of her lost narrative reminds the reader of her complex position in the current narrative; she fills a gap between the omniscient narrator who must remain outside of the plot and a secondary character who has (or had) the potential to generate a plot of her own. The invalid's status, in this case, converts not only her desire for marriage but also the narrative's desire for a marriage plot into her authority to observe and guide.[42]

Martineau reemphasizes Maria's power by ending the novel from within Maria's perspective. Three days before Margaret leaves Deerbrook to marry Enderby, she and Maria sit "by the window, whence they loved to look abroad upon the meadow, wood, and stream" (596). After waiting roughly five hundred pages for this marriage, we end with a slightly unexpected meditation on the future of Maria Young. Although Maria is physically well at the moment, we learn from an earlier scene that her "health is bad" and that she "cannot expect to be able to work always" (296). Margaret tells Maria that only one thing mars her happy ending—that Maria is "infirm and suffering in body, poor, solitary, living in toil, without love, without prospect" (598). Maria rejects Margaret's reminder and the narrator's claims about her condition, asking, "Why we should demand that one lot . . . be as happy as another" (599) and why hers should be like Margaret's. Maria's alignment with the narrator throughout allows us, at this point, to read her assertion about different "lots" not simply as a sign of resignation or stoicism but as a comment on the limitations of certain plot structures, especially for women. While we have been asked periodically to see as Maria does—or at least to notice the differences between Maria's perspective and that of the other characters—the bulk of the novel encourages our identification with Margaret and the marriage plot. In the last few pages, however, Martineau asks us to question the well-worn narrative paths we have come to expect. We are asked at this moment to identify with the power of omniscience—to see in it an ideal condition, a version of health that rivals the heroine's romance. Maria goes on to explain to Margaret that "[i]f you could, for one day and night, feel with my feelings and see through my eyes . . . you would know . . . that there are glimpses of heaven for me in solitude, as for you in love" (599). While critics routinely note the religious overtones of Maria's request, they fail to recognize how such a statement deviates from traditional plots and closure and paves the way for Martineau's turn as an invalid narrator.

Part of this critical inattention comes from the fact that Martineau wraps Maria in the shroud of the redundant woman. Maria's friendship with Margaret often makes her seem as though she is the heroine's uncanny double, but the moments in the novel that identify the invalid with the narrator are moments in which Maria transcends her social role and becomes, instead, a function of narrative. This alternative role for the invalid, as we have seen, becomes more developed as Martineau writes about her own experience. In *Life in the Sick-Room,* Martineau echoes Maria Young's philosophy, explaining, "It is for the interests of truth and temper to remind the healthy and busy . . . that there may be influences in the life of the meditative invalid which may render his views more comprehensive, and his judgments more, rather than less, sound than heretofore" (118). She further argues, "The sufferer may well be satisfied, and needs be abashed before no mortal, if he obtains, sooner or later, the power to achieve divine ends through the experience of his *lot*" (123, emphasis added). Maria makes a claim for equality, while Martineau asserts a kind of superiority; both define their perspectives, their "lots," against the normal to assert, at least narratively, a form of health. And while the audiences for these two texts may be different, both hear the same counsel and the same intense tone—Maria's capacity to "see glimpses of heaven" and the Invalid's ability "to achieve divine ends" become the dividing line between those in the plot and those outside it, between the ordinary and the invalid.

As the ultraobservant and speculative friend with no traditional plot of her own, the invalid should function as a neutral character through which to filter a story. But as we have seen, the condition of invalidism, just like the condition of narration, is anything but neutral, and the privileges of this kind of omniscience come at some cost. Martineau hints at some of the problems with the invalid's privilege in *Life in the Sick-Room.* In a chapter entitled "Some of the Perils and Pains of Invalidism," Martineau warns that "[w]e [invalids] are in ever-growing danger of becoming too abstract—of losing our sympathy with passing emotions" (136) and that too much self-consciousness can lead to false perception (145). These concerns are presented as a caution to invalids—to "the initiated"—so that they may manage their condition and achieve their potential. Such caveats would lead later to Martineau's reevaluation of her "little volume."

In her *Autobiography,* written more than ten years after *Life in the Sick-Room,* she notes that if she were to write *Life* again, she "should have a very different tale to tell" (450). Although she would still "swear" to the "facts . . . and practical doctrine," Martineau was embarrassed by what she describes as "the magnifying of my own experience, the desperate concern as to my own ease and happiness, the moaning undertone running through what many people have called the stoicism, and the total inability to distinguish between the metaphysically apparent and the positively true" (450). It would, she claims, have been better to write a strictly "pathological" study, a kind of medical report for the benefit of science rather than a treatise on the pleasure and value of suffering (432).[43]

But Martineau did not tell a different tale—she did not write a medical manual—and the one she told was tied very much to novelistic fiction; her tale reflects the role that stasis, solitude, and sight play in the construction of the invalid's condition and thus in the production of narrative intelligence. In both texts, Martineau expects her readers to believe in the "peculiar privileges" and the healthy perspective of the invalid that nobody else, except perhaps the narrator in a novel, enjoys. This idealized sense of authority—this access to truth and clear vision—marks the invalid as the stable and necessary observer. Martineau's invalid, like others who resemble her, represents the fantasy of being an omniscient body, perched between presence and absence, insight and foresight, connectedness and isolation. The invalid narrator exposes a range of desires, both social and narrative, that generate plot but also threaten to disrupt it. As such, this figure is not an anomalous kind of narrator but in some ways representative of the way that telling a healthy story and achieving a happy ending may, indeed, be two very different things.

Three

Professionalization

Chapter Five

Narrative Competence and the Family Doctor in Gaskell's *Wives and Daughters*

While the "Rules of Health" are, as George Cheyne states in *Essay of Health and Long Life* (1724), "self-evident," knowing how best to follow them is not. For although one might be familiar with these rules, he is, as the medical literature suggests, often inclined to ignore them—or, worse, "wantonly transgresseth" them, which, according to Cheyne, is "a Degree of Self-Murder."[1] Indeed, medical writers necessarily criticized their readers for focusing on the wrong thing—on cures rather than preventives, on diagnosis at the expense of maintenance. If not for such wrongs, these writers would have had little to teach. But as I have been suggesting, medical advice not only relies for its authority on this lapse, and on its superior knowledge of the body and the burgeoning science of medicine, but also turns to the art of telling stories as a way of convincing readers how best to keep well, how to read for health. William Buchan and Thomas Beddoes created narratives (case studies and fictionalized anecdotes) about neglectful parents, ailing children, and bad readers; Thomas Southwood Smith imagined a doctor's risk of infection to make a point about avoiding epidemic disease. The doctor's expertise, though authorized by his education and professional affiliation, was determined as well by his ability to tell a convincing story and by his capacity to listen to and interpret the stories of his patients. He must recognize the role that the patient's narrative plays, not only in the diagnosis of her symptoms but also in the treatment of her disease and the maintenance of her health.[2]

Storytelling, as the previous chapters imply, is integral to the practice of medicine, and this chapter focuses on the doctor's role not only in shaping the ways Victorians told their stories but also in learning to become competent readers of those stories. Other critics have noted that the doctor-hero was an invention of the nineteenth century.[3] Beginning with Harriet Martineau's Dr. Hope, and finding perhaps its finest representation in the tragic story of George Eliot's Tertius Lydgate, the doctor emerges in novelistic fiction as a socially respectable and narratively desirable figure, valuable both as a bridge between the professional and domestic worlds and as the arbiter of a narrative of public and private health. The first fictional doctor-hero, Martineau's Dr. Hope, endures personal and professional difficulty, as he strives throughout *Deerbrook* to conquer his desire for his wife's sister and to regain his social standing and his income after voting against the village's wealthy patrons in a local election. The townsfolk condemn his new medical ways out of ignorance but eventually praise his efforts after he works tirelessly to save and comfort his neighbors and former patients during a deadly epidemic.

Thirty-some years after *Deerbrook*, Eliot created Tertius Lydgate; by that time, the doctor was no longer considered an inappropriate romantic hero, a mere "medicinal lover," one who, as Sydney Smith claims in an early review of *Deerbrook*, "if [Dr. Hope] takes his mistress's hand with the utmost fervor of a lover, . . . [he] will, by mere force of habit, end in feeling her pulse."[4] But Lydgate suffers domestically because he chooses the wrong wife and professionally because he ignores the power of status quo medical practice. Other characters distrust him because he gets involved in the wrong kind of story. Unlike Hope, however, Lydgate is never rewarded for his troubles. Instead of becoming the scientific pioneer and medical reformer he showed the promise of becoming, Lydgate ends his days administering to the needs of gouty patients in a wealthy spa town. In both cases, the conflict surrounding the medical profession during the early part of the century does not just provide a backdrop for these novelists but also gives shape and depth to the romance plots around which these novels are built. The conflict between the personal and the professional, the domestic and the medical, drives our narrative interests.

During those thirty-three years separating Hope and Lydgate appears Mr. Gibson, the doctor-protagonist of Elizabeth Gaskell's *Wives and Daughters* (1865).[5] Unlike these other fictional doctors, this one has a professional life utterly void of competition and intrigue, which makes him—or should make him—an ideal reader.[6] Mr. Gibson's most pressing medical problem is that he is too good. He is not only an excellent practitioner but also a preeminent educator. The narrator explains that the "prohibitory" fees he charges his new students in the hopes of deterring them from seeking his guidance are "willingly paid, in order that [such] young m[e]n might make a start in life, with the prestige of having been a pupil of Gibson of Hollingford" (33). The professional uncertainty and financial hardships with which characters such as Lydgate and Hope must contend never enter *Wives and Daughters* directly. In fact, with its focus on the love plots of the doctor's daughter, Molly Gibson, and her stepsister, Cynthia Kirkpatrick, *Wives and Daughters* seems hardly to concern itself centrally with the professional conflicts of a village doctor. This is not because Gaskell is unfamiliar with these struggles—her short story "Mr. Harrison's Confessions" deals precisely with the problems a young general practitioner faces when attempting to enact a reforming agenda in a world suspicious of new methods.[7] That nobody questions Mr. Gibson's medical authority, however, does not mean it escapes scrutiny. He may not experience political pressure from outside the home, but Mr. Gibson must contend with the challenges waged from within it; for while Mr. Gibson is an excellent manager of health, he is less adept at telling stories and even more deficient when it comes to listening to them. He needs help, which Gaskell gives him in the form of a daughter. Thus, two elements that occur in tandem in other chapters of this project—preserving health and telling stories—get put to the test in a new and revealing formation in *Wives and Daughters*.

Any question of the doctor's expertise comes not from his peers, pupils, or patients but from his daughter, a character whom we expect to need rather than to appropriate the tools of her father's trade. Molly Gibson does both. She does get sick (like any good heroine must), but her illness is subordinated to the medical education that teaches her to manage the plots of others and to avoid becoming the center of one herself. *Wives and Daughters* thus exemplifies the intricate layering of the hygienic and therapeutic plots that are perhaps more realistic than those from earlier chapters. Unlike her doctor-father, Molly develops a keen understanding of the complex social dynamics among men and women, fathers and daughters, doctors and mothers, that contribute to one's health and to the development of one's story.

Growing up a happy girl in a peaceable kingdom, with a well-respected father and friends who love her, Molly Gibson does not, at first, appear to need a doctor. She awakens in the novel to a world of expectation and the excitement of attending her first gala. As she looks out her window, she is thankful that "it will be a fine day!" for she was afraid "it never never would come; or that if it ever came, it would be a rainy day!" (6). The gratitude and excitement, however, cannot be sustained. Once at the party, she becomes fatigued, overheated, and hungry; she wanders into a strange garden, falls asleep, and must be saved. Hyacinth "Clare" Kirkpatrick, her would-be rescuer and the woman who will become her stepmother, demonstrates little interest in her well-being, however. In fact, she eats the food that has been sent to revive the "[p]oor dear" (18), invents a story about Molly's overeating, and forgets about the girl completely. In such a manner, Gaskell introduces readers to the type of improper management with which Molly must contend; it is such mismanagement she learns to revise throughout the novel. Realizing that Molly has been left by her chaperones at the party, the father-doctor arrives on the scene to take her home, prompting readers to assume that they can relax their vigilant care. All seems to be well again, as Molly promises never to leave her father's side. But then the novel begins again, giving us a second version of the daughter's need for care—and a second version of what proper doctoring might be.

The second beginning—the one in which "the real story of the novel begins"[8]—occurs five years and four chapters later. This time, the doctor must confront his daughter's desirability and the problems that come with romance and intrigue: Molly, at "nearly seventeen," becomes the unwitting heroine of a clandestine romance plot (53). Mr. Gibson intercepts a love letter intended for Molly. As a young woman, the Molly of this second introduction requires an even more watchful eye, her plot becoming even more intertwined with her father's profession, for while she is not yet physically ill, her healthy and maturing female body portends the kind of malady—"love sickness"—that her father fears but that readers so enjoy: Mr. Gibson is "startled into discovering that his little one was growing fast into a woman and already the passive object of some strong interests that affect a woman's life" (55). As in so many novels, healthy female sexuality has to be managed as disease. In response to this social and biological reality, Mr. Gibson sends his daughter away, isolating her from these "interests" that will soon affect her life and have already affected her story. Molly Gibson may not have been "forgotten" as in the first chapter when she is left in the garden, but the type of preventative care she receives has a similar effect: she becomes the focus of the narrative's attention and anxiety, in no small part because her doctor-father's diagnosis of her situation, and the "quarantine" he imposes, leads to her removal from its potentially harmful center.

Having been trained in novelistic medicine as well as in the novel's love-plot formulas, however, we know that by isolating Molly to prohibit contact, the doctor cannot stop the narrative's progress. In fact, this removal does the opposite, creating the time and space for an "interesting" story to develop. Molly's case seems, at first, to fulfill these narrative expectations. Her father sends her to Hamley Hall to visit the invalid Mrs. Hamley at a time when the two eligible sons of the house will be away. While Molly's father and Mrs. Hamley's husband are, for different reasons, glad of this fact, the repeated assurances that there will be *no* romance at Hamley Hall suggest that this is precisely where Molly will find love. And, of course, she does, but not before Gaskell's narrative takes an extended detour that removes Molly from romantic attention and instead frames the heroine's story within the doctor's plot of expertise and education, taking on the role of medical practitioner.

The kind of heroine Molly will come to represent is, at its core, a medical one, for while her own story fits, at least initially, into a hygienic model of narrative (one focused on maintenance and prevention rather than cure), the stories she manages are largely therapeutic; they involve diagnosis, treatment, cure, and death. The medicalization of Molly's plot does not mean, however, that the daughter will simply adopt the doctor-father's authority and reject the stepmother's false stories, which range from little white lies to dangerous plotting; nor does it mean that Molly will be subsumed by her nascent professionalism and removed from future romance altogether.[9] Her brand of medicine, while feminized as sororal or maternal and depicted as an antidote to her stepmother's domestic (mis)management, offers an alternative to her father's paternalistic dosing. The daughter synthesizes and reimagines the two forms of care—the medical and the domestic—in terms of their shared dependence on narrative competence. Molly not only must learn to, as physician and medical educator Rita Charon has recently suggested in reference to medical training in narrative, "absorb, interpret, and respond to stories"[10] but also must become the author of her own story. In offering medicine as a cure for the romantic interests that interfere with but also sustain domestic health, Gaskell articulates a version of medicine that must be attentive to stories and to narrative.[11] To be a doctor means more than being a practitioner of medicine or a taker of pulses; it means combining the lessons of domestic fiction with the teachings of scientific discovery to produce (with the patient) a healthy body and a healthy narrative.

MEDICAL PRACTICE: THE DOCTOR

Gaskell initially signals the importance of the doctor's professional history to her heroine's story by embedding it in the novel's structure; she fills the time and space between Molly's two introductions with the story of Mr. Gibson's rise as the town's doctor.[12] The chapter that tells us about Molly Gibson's childhood does not begin when Molly is born or even when her parents first meet; it takes place "[s]ixteen years before [the gala]" (29) with Mr. Gibson's ascension as the town's new doctor. The narrator describes the moment when Mr. Gibson moves into Hollingford as a "disturb[ance]" for the town's citizens (29). Mr. Hall, we are told, "'slyly' . . . introduce[s] [Mr. Gibson] into practice" (30). A sense of harmless deception and a disruption to the status quo surrounds the doctors' partnership, qualities that will become increasingly important to Molly's development. Mr. Hall is too old and too sick to fulfill his duties, but his patients are suspicious of newcomers and new ways. As "blind and deaf, and rheumatic as he might be," we are told, "he was still Mr. Hall, the doctor who could heal all their ailments—unless they died meanwhile—and had no right to speak of growing old, and taking a partner" (30). Gaskell's portrait of the power of the desire of patients and the friendly conflict between old and new medicine adds verisimilitude to the story, but it depicts as well the kind of fluidity that allowed for change and innovation in medical practice to occur. While Mr. Gibson's gentility and mysterious lineage appeal to the townspeople, his professional ability helps "the younger doctor carr[y] the day" (31). Within a year of his arrival, he becomes the preferred partner, earning the respect of Sir Astley (president of the College of Surgeons) and the patronage of "the Towers" (31). Mr. Gibson lodges us firmly in the world of expertise and talent—his cutting-edge training in Edinburgh and Paris and his professional ethics are beyond reproach.[13]

Even with the right education, the right credentials, and the right looks, however, Mr. Gibson (we soon learn) lacks the right kind of narrative competence—or rather, he lacks the capacity to see, as Molly eventually does, that doctoring is as much a narrative endeavor as it is a clinical practice. Gaskell eases the reader into this narrative view of medical practice with an early scene that uses the written prescription as a vehicle of its satire. As with medical manuals and reports, a prescription holds out the promise, potentially a guarantee, of health, though in some cases it can only offer mild comfort. Regardless of its outcome, the prescription is an instruction, generally written, that tells the patient how to achieve or maintain health. Mr. Gibson is, we presume, an expert prescriber, knowing precisely which drafts and doses to offer. In this instance, however, he uses the prescription to perform a textual joke. After intercepting a "flaming love-letter" from his apprentice, Mr. Coxe, to his daughter, Mr. Gibson interprets its contents as symptomatic of illness—"[c]alf-love," he calls it—and responds to it by writing a supposed cure. He sends the "patient" the follow prescription (50):

> Rx Verecundiae ʒ i.
> Fidelitatis Domesticae ʒ i.
> Reticentiae gr. iij.
> M. Capiat hanc dosim ter die in aquâ purâ.
>
> R. GIBSON, *Ch*

Modesty, domestic fidelity, and deference, mixed with pure water and taken three times a day, will, Mr. Gibson jokes, cure the ailment.

This mock prescription is designed to humiliate the suitor and thwart Molly's love plot, and although it is not a real prescription, it does act as a curative agent; it obstructs the lover's and the reader's (if she does not speak Latin) momentum and delays Molly's entrance into the traditional story of romance and marriage. Rather than speak to Mr. Gibson as a frustrated suitor, Mr. Coxe accepts the metaphor upon which the joke relies and allows the doctor-patient performance to continue, leading Mr. Gibson further down the path of metaphorical doctoring. Mr. Coxe objects to the treatment, but the doctor claims, "[P]atients are sometimes offended at being told the nature of their illnesses; and, I dare say, they may take offence at the medicine which their case requires" (52). Though we know from his history that Mr. Gibson is a respected doctor, Gaskell begins to challenge his authority here, for he is only playing doctor when it comes to domestic matters of romantic affection. Though playfulness is certainly in order, Gaskell exposes a slippage between the medical and the romantic; and Mr. Gibson's discomfort with negotiating successfully between the two modes opens the narrative and recuperative/healer's space that Molly will fill.

The prescription may stave off infection, but it does little to halt the narrative's desire to move Molly into the realm of romance. And although Mr. Gibson is a "clever surgeon" (33), he appears here to be an ineffectual practitioner of domestic management, which is not to say that he is a bad doctor or father. The novel represents him as superior in both respects. But his misreading of Molly, his surprise that Mr. Coxe wants to woo his daughter, and his ineffectual appropriation of medical metaphors speak to a deficiency in his ability to read and interpret the narratives of domestic life and domestic medicine. This gap in his knowledge and inattentiveness cannot be filled by a traditional or even fictional prescription. Upon learning of Molly's desirability, Mr. Gibson reasons with himself that she cannot be an object of desire because "she is only just seventeen—not seventeen, indeed, till July; not for six weeks. Sixteen and three-quarters! Why she is quite a baby" (49). He describes Molly in terms that do not quite match her chronological age, calling her "a mere child" (52), even though we know from the narrator that her childhood is over, neatly contained within a single chapter. For a doctor, whose ability is to see the body in ways others cannot, this is not a good sign. Mr. Gibson ignores Mr. Coxe's rejoinder that "Miss Gibson is nearly seventeen! I heard you say so only the other day" (53), holding to the argument that such clandestine behavior violates "the laws of domestic honour" (52). The doctor's insistence on keeping Molly a child exposes both his professional and his paternal fallibility, particularly when it comes to interpreting the signs of romance. Only at the end of the novel, when Molly's physical health is endangered, does he regain his authority over her as a medical doctor. For now, because she has always been his little "Goosey," he is "startled" by Molly's womanhood in a way that we assume a mother would not have been. With her governess away, taking care of a nephew with scarlet fever, and a father who must be away from home attending to his patients, Molly is left unguided and vulnerable to romantic overtures. Instead of talking to Molly about the letter or his concern about her safety and thus inoculating her against future advances, he sends her away—in full health and because she is in full health—to buy some time to find the right preventive.

Precisely when she is removed from her father's sphere, she begins to develop a sense of domestic medicine that will prove to challenge her father's supposedly stable authority as a practitioner. Molly's entrance into Hamley Hall protects her from a premature engagement or, perhaps worse, the anxiety of having to refuse a suitor—but more than that, it educates her in the forces that affect personal and family health. For while the novel has thus far been motivated by the desire to maintain Molly's health, its energies shift now into developing Molly's interest in the stories of others. The doctoring hero turns out to be the daughter after all, and Hamley becomes an important training ground for her apprenticeship, as she begins to learn how the desire for—and loss of—health shapes the narratives of those around her. Up to this point in the novel,

Gaskell has afforded Mr. Gibson qualified authority as a doctor. By relocating Molly in the sickly household, however, Gaskell begins to transfer control of the story and of the medicine from the doctor to his daughter, and what seemingly better place to isolate Molly from romance and introduce her to the world of doctoring than the home of an invalid wife? Molly is transformed in this environment from a heroine-in-waiting to an apprentice-in-training, as this temporary home teaches her about marriage, medicine, and the value of narrative authority to both.

But Molly must first learn what it means to be a wife and a mother, two components of domesticity absent from her upbringing. Because Molly's mother died when she was a child, she has not witnessed the relationship between husband and wife—the Hamleys provide her with her first experience of this matrimonial bond. But the kind of marriage and maternal care she encounters is sickly. Mrs. Hamley's invalidism, we are told by the narrator, is a result of her marriage to the squire. Any sense of a romantic past we might imagine for this husband and wife is overtly pathologized. Marriage, family, and illness are of a piece in this home. It is true that Mrs. Hamley had been a "delicate fine London lady" before meeting the Squire, but this alone does not account for her current invalidism (42). In the same breath we are told that Squire and Mrs. Hamley are "very happy" together and that "possibly Mrs. Hamley would not have sunk into the condition of a chronic invalid, if her husband had cared a little more for her various tastes, or allowed her the companionship of those who did" (42). The narrator's speculation that Mr. Hamley's insecurities contributed to his wife's condition, though not an endorsement of matrimony, seems less a critique of marriage and more a commentary on a particular match. Theirs was "one of those perplexing marriages of which one cannot understand the reason" (42). The Squire is "awkward and ungainly," "obstinate, violent-tempered, and dictatorial," but he is also "generous, and true as steel," something Mr. Gibson, as our initial arbiter of good character, observes—he likes the Squire, and that is enough to make us accept Mr. Hamley's marriage to a woman who is a "great reader" and "literary," as well as "gentle and sentimental; tender and good" (42). Her willingness to "sacrific[e]" her social and intellectual life, though ultimately fatal, makes the Squire "lov[e] his wife more dearly" (42). And for that we might forgive him.

At first, Mrs. Hamley's story invokes a common use of illness within the marriage plot, wherein the suffering female spouse is sickly, frail, or an invalid. Critics have observed that Molly learns about pathological womanhood in this setting.[14] With Mrs. Hamley, we witness, according to the doctor, "real secret harm" and "growing and indescribable discomfort" (43). And although her illness resists a specific diagnosis—it is "nothing definite"—Gaskell is quick to assert that Mrs. Hamley was not "merely [a] fanciful invalid" (44). Mr. Gibson hoped that by "careful watching of her symptoms he might mitigate her bodily pain" (44). Her body, however, resists a permanent cure, and the narrator proposes the daughter as an alternative. "Perhaps if [Mrs. Hamley] had had a daughter," we are told, "it would have been better for her" (43). It is too late for this, and Molly appears in the wake of the sympathetic doctor as the salve for a sickly marriage and an invalid wife.

Molly's apprenticeship, however, involves more than expressing daughterly affection or nursely care; Mrs. Hamley's invalidism is not designed simply to register the toll of living in a patriarchal society. Rather, the role Mrs. Hamley fills so well is that of the storyteller. Molly must learn from the invalid's privileged perspective what health looks like before she can engage in any doctoring of her own. And invalidism in this instance is, for Gaskell, emblematic of the kind of authority and control afforded to narrators; following in the tradition set by Harriet Martineau and others, Gaskell imagines that genuine pain, and the stasis to which it gives rise, is the foundation for a kind of guiding power. As Gaskell demonstrates in *Round the Sofa* (1859), a collection of previously published short stories, the "crippled" Mrs. Dawson is simultaneously at center stage and on the sidelines. Gaskell connects the various tales in this collection by framing them as part of an invalid's entertainment, a break in the "monotony of the nights." Invalidism becomes the source and cause of narration—if not for Mrs. Dawson, neither stories nor narrative would exist. We see this potential in Mrs. Hamley, and although she does not reflect the kind of assertiveness, omniscience, or healthfulness we get from Gaskell's other invalids, she does offer Molly a model for what it means to be simultaneously a teller of stories and a listener. This position (and the ability to move between these roles) becomes a marker of Molly's domesticated medical practice and the sympathy, compassion, and attentiveness that define it.

It is not that Molly learns to mimic Mrs. Hamley or even idolize her. In fact, Mrs. Hamley's perspective is faulty and quite dangerous. Rather, what Molly must experience is the power of the story to heal as well as to harm. This is part of her "clinical" training, as it were. We understand early on that

> [t]he greater part of [Mrs. Hamley's] life was spent on a sofa, wheeled to the window in the summer, to the fireside in the winter. The room which she inhabited was large and pleasant; four tall windows looked out upon the lawn dotted over with flower-beds, and melting away into a small wood, in the centre of which there was a pond, filled with water-lilies. About this unseen pond in the deep shade Mrs. Hamley had written many a pretty four-versed poem since she lay on her sofa, alternately reading and composing poetry. (44)

Highlighting the artistic facets of Mrs. Hamley's identity, and setting her up as a detached observer, looking out the window from her sofa, Gaskell nonetheless does not give this ailing woman the "clear-sightedness" that other invalids in this study possess. Mrs. Hamley is blind to the character of her eldest son, Osborne, a fact that lulls Molly into thinking he is "his mother's hero" (81). His failure at school, his inability to earn a living as a poet, and, we learn eventually, his secret marriage are a far cry from the story

Mrs. Hamley tells about her delicate, clever, and beloved son. This view of Osborne contrasts implicitly with her loving but certainly not so adulatory perspective of her second son, the robust, practical, natural scientist, Roger Hamley.

The role of observer, and the authority that comes with the invalid's perspective, gets dispersed in Gaskell's novel; part of it is given initially to the doctor, who can diagnose "real pain" and catch would-be suitors in the act, and part of it is given to the daughter, who develops the powers of subtle narrative understanding that the novel values more than the doctor's diagnostic skills. Susan Morgan attributes Molly's superior doctoring to her expressiveness and to her "warm, loving heart."[15] These attributes, coupled with her "effort and sense," allow her to excel in her father's field.[16] "The real doctor," as Morgan asserts, "is, of course, Molly."[17] What links Mr. Gibson to his daughter, I am arguing—or rather, what puts them in competition—has to do with the different ways they understand and use narrative in medicine. Not only does Molly develop her sympathy through contact with the invalid, but also she develops a keen awareness of the role that stories play in comfort, treatment, and health.

By constructing the relationship between narrative competence and proper doctoring through Molly's interactions with Mrs. Hamley and invalidism, Gaskell offers a version of care that relies on telling and listening to stories. But it is not until Molly returns to Hamley later in the novel that we begin to see her doctoring abilities more clearly. Her initial visit introduces her to this practice, but we see later in the novel how she puts it to use. Mrs. Hamley's health eventually deteriorates once she learns the truth about the failings of her son Osborne and internalizes the conflict this causes in the family—Squire Hamley will not speak to Osborne. Mr. Gibson has already been to see Mrs. Hamley after this revelation and the downward turn of her health, but only when the daughter returns do we see a truly domestic medicine at work. The Squire announces Molly, noting that "the doctor's daughter [is] nearly as good as the doctor himself" (190). As if taking this cue, Molly assesses her patient's symptoms: the narrator explains that "even with Molly's small experience of illness she saw how much of restless fever there was in [the invalid's] speech; and instinct, or some such gift, prompted [Molly] to tell a long story of many things" (190). "Telling a long story" (the content of which is irrelevant) is not a diagnostic tool or a cure—the patient does not reveal the cause of her complaint through her story. Rather, the story provides comfort, as Molly has a "gift," a kind of vocational talent, for knowing the value of such an act, something her father's medicine, which focuses on therapeutics (prescriptions), does not quite acknowledge. The daughter's presence cannot save Mrs. Hamley, but contact with the invalid has allowed Molly to learn how stories work and that they matter, both to the doctor and to her own plot.

DOMESTIC (MIS)MANAGEMENT: THE MOTHER

At the same time that Molly undergoes her apprenticeship with the Hamleys, her father takes pains to fortify his home for her return. If his wife (Molly's stepmother), Hyacinth "Clare" Kirkpatrick, is not precisely the opposite of Mrs. Hamley, she certainly represents an alternative version of mother, doctor, and storyteller. Both women engage in deceptive narrative practices. Mrs. Hamley creates a romance about Osborne that precipitates both of their tragic ends, whereas Hyacinth tells endless, adulterated tales about herself and her daughter, Cynthia Kirkpatrick, that get the mother in trouble. We see a glimpse of this propensity in the small lie she tells about the eating habits of young Molly in the opening segment (chapter 2). By marrying the doctor to a woman whom Molly calls a "plotter," Gaskell instantiates a tension between medicine and storytelling that the heroine and the reader will learn to negotiate.

We have seen Mr. Gibson's flawed domestic management when he refuses to read Molly's sexual age, yet we accept this bit of parental amnesia because even the most loving of fathers often refuse to see their daughters as women.[18] But choosing Hyacinth as his wife is a misstep of a different sort. How could he have picked so poorly? And why does Gaskell choose for him to do so? In part, he is desperate. With Molly's governess exposed to scarlet fever and unable to return as chaperone (Molly has never had the disease) and with the recent rebellion of his servants, Mr. Gibson has no one left to oversee his domestic affairs. A visit from Lord Hollingford becomes "the final drop—the last straw" that convinces Mr. Gibson to find a second wife. When the fellow widowers sit down to lunch at Mr. Gibson's house, the disorder is too noticeable to avoid comment. The lunch is delayed, the dishes are dirty, and the servants are sulky. The doctor explains, "You see a man like me—a widower—with a daughter who cannot always be at home—has not the regulated household which would enable me to command the small portions of time I can spend there" (101). The dashes in his speech betray a discomfort and hesitancy that we have not previously seen in Mr. Gibson and that we would not expect from our doctor. Hollingford offers the remedy in the form of a second marriage: "If you found a sensible agreeable woman of thirty or so, I really think you couldn't do better than to take her to manage your home, and so save you the discomfort or worry; and besides, she would be able to give your daughter the kind of tender supervision which, I fancy, all girls of that age require" (101). When presented in this light—more as a job for hire—Mr. Gibson wastes no time setting about the business of getting a second wife to manage his home.

From our first introduction to Hyacinth—that day she finds Molly ailing but eats her food—we know she will be a bad mother, even though she does appear to be an astute manager of her own self-interest. Even as it holds Mrs. Gibson up as a negative example, the novel cannot deny her abilities as a social and household manager. Elizabeth Langland offers a recuperative reading of Hyacinth, claiming that to "interpret [her] negatively" is to miss Gaskell's social critique. I agree with Langland that Mrs. Gibson is "a social mentor who makes the doctor and his daughter figures to be reckoned with socially."[19] Mrs. Gibson's successes in the present narrative are built on the failures of the past. Reading hygienically—that is, as a preventionist—we recognize that she has dangerously, almost tragically, mismanaged her own daughter's childhood, something with which Gaskell was deeply concerned, as I discuss below in reference to her diary. The reader knows (and Mr. Gibson must learn) that his wife has her own interests, her own story to tell, which will very quickly conflict with the doctor's and with Molly's and has already conflicted with those of her daughter, Cynthia. She offers a decidedly unhealthy narrative of domestic and maternal nurturance.

We witness, before Molly does, Mrs. Gibson's management of Cynthia, which prepares readers for the preventive stance Molly must take in relation to her stepmother. When Mr. Gibson provides the necessary money to bring Cynthia home for the wedding, Hyacinth Kirkpatrick (soon to be Mrs. Gibson), temporarily moved by this gesture and the funds, imagines that she wishes Cynthia to be a bridesmaid. However, as the narrator explains,

> a hundred little interruptions came in the way of letter-writing; and by the next day maternal love had diminished; and the value affixed to the money had increased: money had been so much needed, so hardly earned in Mrs. Kirkpatrick's life; while the perhaps necessary separation of mother and child had lessened the amount of affection the former had to bestow. (140)

Financial and domestic necessities cannot always accommodate maternal affection. Absence and limited funds, it seems, do not make the heart grow fonder. Not only does Hyacinth wish to keep her attractive daughter away from the wedding, but also she wants to use the money intended to bring Cynthia home to pay her debts and buy gowns that will impress the Hollingford ladies. The narrator acknowledges that Hyacinth's financial fastidiousness is a credit to her otherwise "superficial and flimsy character" (140), but it comes at a price for the daughter, whose inability to pay her own debt creates the central problem to be solved before the novel's end, the problem that will become Molly's greatest case. By filling the vital role of domestic manager with a neglectful and unobservant mother, Gaskell thus creates the necessary condition for Molly's ascension and for the rise of a domestic medicine not only in Mr. Gibson's home but also in the novel more generally. In the form of Hyacinth, the person who is supposed to mitigate future sickness and preserve health—the mother—becomes the very person who creates the "dis-ease" that can cause physical and psychological illness.

Through the presence of Cynthia Kirkpatrick, Gaskell begins to establish Molly, rather than Cynthia's mother or Molly's father, as the superior domestic manager and doctor. When Mrs. Gibson offhandedly refers to Cynthia as "poor dear," Molly thinks immediately of Cynthia's health: why else would a mother call her daughter "a poor dear"? Mrs. Gibson assures her that the "poor" refers to her status as "a fatherless girl" and that "Cynthia never is ill. She's as strong as a horse" (214). Mrs. Gibson does not fear for her daughter's well-being in the way Molly expects a mother might, worrying instead about her own health and comfort. When mother and daughter reunite, Mrs. Gibson comments simply that Cynthia has grown and "look[s] quite a woman"; Cynthia reminds her mother that she has "hardly grown since" she went away and that, in appearance at least, she is relatively the same (215). Later, however, when Miss Hornblower (an acquaintance from Ashcombe) sees Cynthia for the first time in two or three years, she, too, observes, "How she has grown!" (283). Thus we see that Cynthia, in fact, has denied the truth of her mother's statement: she has "grown," but she cannot abide the perfunctoriness of her mother's greeting, a greeting that any Miss Hornblower might give.

Such faulty observations combined with blind confidence in her daughter's health mark Mrs. Gibson as a bad mother. In this novel, bad mothers are bad storytellers and even worse listeners. Cynthia criticizes her mother for "invent[ing] stories" (346, 374), and until she comes to Hollingford and can represent herself, Cynthia's narrative must be filtered through her mother; Cynthia is, as Hilary Schor explains, "introduced through her mother's accounts, her character suggested through her mother's inattention."[20] But from very early on, Molly demonstrates the desire to manage Cynthia's narrative, to take on her "case," attempting to extricate her story from Hyacinth's. During Molly's first extended conversation with her father's fiancée, prior to the wedding, she asks about the daughter who is to come and live with them: "When will she come?"; "When will she leave school?"; "Is she like you?"; "Is she very clever and accomplished?" (128–29). Far from providing satisfying answers, Hyacinth's responses redirect the conversation to her own concerns: "I don't think I must let her leave before next summer"; "She is very handsome, people say. In the bright-coloured style—perhaps something like I was"; "She ought to be [clever and accomplished]; I've paid ever so much money" (128–29). Mrs. Gibson refuses to give over the narrative to her daughter—the "She" must always defer to the "I," as the mother continually thinks in terms of her own interests, comfort, and story.

The proper relationship between mothering and doctoring is, for Gaskell, both personal and fundamental to her own development as a writer. In *My Diary: The Early Years of My Daughter Marianne*, the journal she began keeping in 1835 shortly after the birth of her daughter, Gaskell describes the tremendous work that goes into maintaining good (or at least moderate) health.[21] From it, we get a sense of the pleasure one feels when health has been maintained or achieved, as well as the pleasure one feels when writing about that success. Gaskell begins her first entry by remarking that she wished she had begun the journal sooner because Marianne has already given her so much to write about; she is becoming "every day more and more interesting."[22] Mr. Gibson finds "interest" in his pubescent daughter something to fear, whereas Gaskell sees it, even in her baby, as the impetus for writing. In fact, in the second entry, written almost five months later, Gaskell laments that she has waited so long to write about her "little darling"; she deems herself "negligent." Here, Gaskell imagines writing to be not only an important duty but also one that, with each passing entry, is increasingly tied to observations about her daughter's health. Throughout, Gaskell turns the reader's attention to Marianne's physical state: she is described variously as "still a delicate child," "a frail little treasure," and "very weak in her limbs" (12, 13, 19). We also learn of the improvements, as when, on February 7, 1836, Gaskell explains, "[Marianne's] whole body bespeaks a more healthy child" and continues, "She has a colour like a cherry, instead of the flushed wavering red it used to be; and certainly with health, beauty comes" (21). These episodes—the shift from the flushed, frail treasure to the cherry-cheeked beauty—shape the story Gaskell wants to tell about her daughter's development and the advice she wants to give her daughter should she ever have a child of her own.

Though the diary is more episodic than novelistic, Gaskell develops her maternal musings and a sense of the value of narrative within and against a larger framework of expert, professional opinion. She complains in one entry that it is difficult to know how to handle her daughter's impatience because "*every body* and every book says that decision is of such consequence" (12). Gaskell finds little comfort in these kinds of child-care "books," which, as she says, "do so differ," but such guides are not the only "books" Gaskell refers to in her diary. For example, she cites Andrew Combe's *Principles of Physiology* as having "prepared" her to understand the relationship between her daughter's "bodily feeling" and her mental temperament. Published in 1834, Combe's book endeavors to teach people how their bodies work and how best to care for them.[23] But instead of deferring to the advice Combe and others offer, Gaskell writes herself into a collaborative partnership with them. She suggests at one point that only through experience, a mother's experience, can one understand fully the relationship between the "temper" and the "body." "Mothers," she explains, "are sometimes laughed at for attributing little freaks of temper to teething, &c., but I don't think those who laugh at them (I used to be one) have had much to do with children" (*Diary*, 14). Her experience and newfound expertise are not subordinate to Combe's; neither are they held out as superior. Later, however, when discussing one of Marianne's various recoveries, Gaskell does begin to introduce her own expert authority more overtly: "With her strength has her good temper returned, which is in accordance with my theory that when *children* . . . are irritable something is physically the matter with them" (*Diary*, 17). Here, Gaskell identifies herself as a theorist among the experts and a manager among doctors. Doctors are not, as the diary suggests, the sole authority on healthy families. And Gaskell's authority comes not only from her status as a mother but also from her narrative competence, which she is developing through the very writing of this diary.

The relationship between mothering and writing transforms in *Wives and Daughters* into a relationship between medical expertise and narrative competence. It is a relationship that Gaskell locates in the figure of the daughter. As a daughter (who is not yet a mother or a wife), Molly inhabits a kind of training ground, suspended in that moment of "interest" when so much is still possible. But rather than offer Molly or the reader an ideal version of the mother-doctor on which to model her behavior, Gaskell presents us with its opposite in Mrs. Gibson. Nowhere do we see the clash between medicine and domestic management more clearly than when Mrs. Gibson overhears her husband discussing Osborne Hamley's medical diagnosis with another physician, Mr. Nicholls. As if eavesdropping on a patient consultation were not enough of an invasion, Mrs. Gibson sneaks in to the surgery to look up the name of Osborne's disease before deciding what kind of advantage it will give her. Up to this point, she has been trying and failing to create a love plot involving Osborne and Cynthia. Not until Mrs. Gibson realizes that he has a fatal illness and that his younger brother, Roger Hamley, is likely to become the heir to the estate does she support the relationship between Roger and Cynthia. When Mrs. Gibson exposes her enthusiasm for the engagement and reveals her knowledge about Osborne's health, Mr. Gibson becomes greatly concerned. A diagnosis, which is only speculative, reached his wife's ears, creating a personal and professional dilemma for the doctor. Mr. Gibson forces his wife to repeat what she overheard, thus turning her into the bearer of Osborne's diagnosis for the reader—it is from her mouth that we hear he has "an aneurism of the aorta" and that "there is a pretty clear indication of symptoms" (381). She recapitulates his diagnosis word for word, such that Mr. Gibson cannot pretend that he was referring to another patient.

Rather than marking a distinction between Mr. Gibson and his wife, this episode aligns the two performers and thus makes way for Molly's form of domestic medicine. When he asks, "How do you know we were speaking of Osborne Hamley?" Hyacinth takes this query as a sign that "he was descending to her level of subterfuge," a shift that gives her more "courage" and a sense of authority to speak (381). The narrator explains that at this moment she takes on "quite a different tone to the cowed one which she had been using" (381). The doctor and his wife speak, if only momentarily, the same language, as it becomes Mr. Gibson's turn to articulate for the reader what Mrs. Gibson has been thinking and doing. He takes on her perspective, surmising that she "made [Roger] more welcome in the house than [she] had ever done before, regarding him as proximate heir to the Hamley estate" (382). When Mrs. Gibson claims not to know the meaning of "proximate," Mr. Gibson retorts, "Go into the surgery, and look in the dictionary then" (382). This spatial and rhetorical breach of public and private, of doctor and wife, marks the limits of how these roles can be traversed. It is not that the mother should not enter the realm of medicine—mothers, as Gaskell's diary demonstrates, are de facto doctors, observing symptoms, making diagnoses, and determining treatment. Rather, it is that Mrs. Gibson uses the expertise of the surgery to draw the wrong kind of conclusions. For her, Osborne's diagnosis is economic rather than medical, and entirely self-interested. Although we know that her "maneuver" has no real authority—Osborne is already secretly married and Cynthia has already accepted Roger's proposal—it functions as a model against which we see Molly cultivate her own connection among medicine, domestic management, and narrative.

DOMESTIC MEDICINE: THE DAUGHTER

While the focus of the plot turns to Cynthia Kirkpatrick's romantic relationships, the novel is ultimately interested in developing Molly's authority through her ability to keep Cynthia morally rather than simply physically healthy. Cynthia's story becomes a way for Molly to assert her expertise.[24] For although Cynthia is "as strong as a horse," Gaskell brings her into the doctor's house to have her cured of her incessant plotting. The person to cure Cynthia is not the clever doctor but the clever doctor's daughter. Like her mother, Cynthia has stories to tell, and if she were in charge of the narrative, this would be a very different novel. When she arrives from boarding school, she brings with her a secret, unwanted engagement, which we do not find out about until much later. For now, she cryptically and teasingly tells Molly that she is "not good, and . . . never shall be," though she leaves room for the possibility that she "might be a heroine still" (221). At one point, she explains that her plan is to become a governess and move to Russia. Set in a foreign land, the story she might invent for herself would center on an English governess who, neglected by her mother and taken advantage of by an older man, never marries. We only get glimpses of this potential narrative, but from early on we are suspicious of Cynthia's threat to abscond to Russia and live as a governess. That is, we are fairly certain that she will never fulfill this promise.

By the time Cynthia comes to live with the Gibsons, Molly, though still innocent, has already learned a great deal about sickness and love stories. Summoned to Hamley to soothe the dying wife, Molly learns that such stories, which seem always to have secrets, can be "very uncomfortable" and that their heroes can be rather disappointing. Molly's apprenticeship has prepared her for Cynthia's secret anxiety, and while the illness in Cynthia's plot is largely metaphorical—she never becomes an invalid like Mrs. Hamley—Gaskell nonetheless stages Cynthia's story as in need of medical intervention. The action of the novel revolves around Molly honing her abilities to read and manage plots, thus delaying or rather disrupting her own entrance into romance and marriage. For although we know that Molly is never truly absent from the plot, by handing the management of Cynthia over to her, Gaskell gives Molly time (and several hundred pages) to become something other than a daughter or a wife—she becomes a manager of health and of stories, which, for Gaskell, is what the daughter must do to become a competent wife and mother.

Molly's skills are put the test with Cynthia. We see the beginnings of her "practice" when Mr. Preston, the man who has extorted an engagement from Cynthia, calls on the Gibsons. As the Cumnor land agent and a friend from Hyacinth's days at Ashcombe, Mr. Preston's attentions are expected and fit well within the bounds of social etiquette. Molly knows Mr. Preston from her father's wedding, and his flirtatious, insincere manners make her uncomfortable and impatient. It is no surprise, then, that when Hyacinth lies to him about Cynthia's whereabouts Molly attempts to participate in deception. Hearing the "click" of the door, Molly realizes that Cynthia has returned and tries to stop her (without any hint from Mrs. Gibson) from entering the room. Molly's dislike for Mr. Preston and her uncharacteristically "maliciou[s] desir[e] to baffle him" aligns her momentarily with Mrs. Gibson. But instead of blocking the encounter, Molly gets tangled up in "crewels of worsted" (226): in effect, Gaskell prohibits her heroine from participating in subterfuge. While Molly is physically incapable of (or too clumsy for) this kind of trickery and intrigue, her thwarted attempt to become a bit of a "plotter" suggests that she will need to offer Cynthia a different form of care than what the mother has provided.

Her aborted effort to stop the encounter between Cynthia and Preston is not simply an example of bad management; it provides Molly with an opportunity to begin her physical examination of Cynthia, to begin using the medical training she developed at Hamley Hall. When Cynthia sees Mr. Preston in her drawing room, the narrator explains, "Her colour, which had been brilliant the first moment of her entrance, faded away as she gazed; but her eyes—her beautiful eyes—usually so soft and grave, seemed to fill with fire" (227). Though we do not yet know the reason for Cynthia's reaction, Mr. Preston's interest in Cynthia is clearly sexual and thus dangerous. The description of Cynthia appears to be focalized through all three characters (Molly, Mr. Preston, and Mrs. Gibson) simultaneously, though with very different meanings. The refrain "her beautiful eyes" is the language of a lover, a sisterly statement of admiration, and a momentary reflection of a mother's pride; the narrator notes that "all were looking at [Cynthia] with different emotions" (227). The additional observation that Cynthia's eyes are "usually so soft and grave" seems to be wholly of Molly's notice (and a product of her diagnostic gaze). As objects of Cynthia's disaffection, Mr. Preston and Mrs. Gibson are rarely on the receiving end of such "softness." Indeed, when Cynthia has a similar physical response later, only Molly questions what it means. As the stepsisters read the too-familiar note Mr. Preston sends to Cynthia, signed only "R.P.," the narrator explains, "Cynthia looked extremely irritated, indignant, perplexed—what was it turned her cheek so pale, and made her eyes so full of fire?" (280). The question and thus the observation is Molly's, and while she has already seen Cynthia turn pale and fire-eyed in the presence of Mr. Preston, she does not connect the man with his initials. This time Cynthia intensifies her symptoms by making them literal, by throwing the flowers—"the remind[er] of that man"—into the fire (280). This event becomes part of the "case history" of Cynthia that Molly implicitly puts together.[25]

Gaskell thus links the sisters' plots by attaching Molly and her diagnostic gaze fully to Cynthia's case. The primary narrative desire underlying the charity ball they attend comes neither from Molly's excitement about its being her first nor from her pleasure at having so many interesting partners. Rather, what drives this episode is Molly's intense commitment to Cynthia's well-being. She is, the narrator explains, "more occupied in watching Cynthia" than in attending to her mother's chastisement. Molly devotes all of her interest to "understand[ing] the change that seemed to have come over" her sister, "nurs[ing]" her "curiosity"—the medical metaphor is telling—"into a very proper desire for further information" (120). Molly notices all the ways in which Cynthia's demeanor changes over the course of the evening: Cynthia exhibits "the same lightness and grace [when she dances], but the smooth bounding motion as of a feather . . . [is] gone"; "she [is] conversing with her partner, but without the soft animation that [is] usually shown upon her countenance"; and finally, she "change[s] colour" and her eyes turn "dreamily abstract" (294). With Molly's visual examination complete, she has enough evidence to ask what is wrong. When Cynthia denies any problem, Molly presents her with the symptoms and tentative diagnosis: "[Y]ou look different to what you did—tired or something" (294). Though she cannot yet figure out the problem—she does not know exactly which questions to ask or how far she should probe—Molly does reveal her nascent competence in domestic medicine. Brought up in a doctor's house, trained as an invalid's confidante, Molly has become skilled in reading bodily signs of distress.

These diagnostic instincts are tested shortly after the ball, when Cynthia becomes mildly indisposed. Her languidness and altered looks during this period are not, as Mrs. Gibson later casts it, attributable to Roger Hamley's absence: they are a direct result of Cynthia's encounter with Mr. Preston. This indisposition is the first physical sign of the seriousness of her secret arrangement, and Mrs. Gibson fails to understand its significance. The narrator compares the mother's and the sister's response to Cynthia's health, explaining that "Mrs. Gibson noticed it" but "Molly became positively uneasy" (311). The sick daughter, who should cause at least some maternal anxiety, only makes Mrs. Gibson "impatient"; she "accuse[s] Cynthia of being fanciful and lazy" (311). Mr. Gibson, partially "at Molly's instance [*sic*]," conducts "a professional examination," which reveals "that there was nothing very much the matter, only a general lowness of tone, and a depression of health and sprits" (311). He offers his patient a prescription, which, as we have seen, is the doctor's standard response: Cynthia can either take a "tonic" or she can talk about the problem. "If you tell me your sorrows and cares," he cajoles, "I'll try to find some other remedy for them than giving you what you are pleased to term my nauseous mixtures" (311). Both options hold the same weight for Mr. Gibson, for even though he agrees to hear her story, it is only for the sake of determining "some other remedy." Cynthia chooses the "nauseous mixtures" without telling her story. As expected, she does not waste away under the anxiety and pressure; she recovers from her "supposed invalid[ism]" (310), and while Mrs. Gibson is right (Cynthia's illness is not serious), the mother's unwillingness to take her daughter more seriously—to hear her story—blinds her to the true cause of her metaphorical disease, a plot at the end of which Cynthia sees only "doom" (329).

The problem with Cynthia's story is not simply that it involves intrigue (something we know is forbidden in the Gibson household) but that it affects Roger. At the same time Molly struggles with Cynthia's mysterious behavior, she must contend with Roger's obvious attachment to Cynthia and with Molly's own growing desire for the young man. Molly is not the only one who observes Cynthia's waning health: "[T]he first person out of the house to notice Cynthia's change of look and manner was Roger Hamley" (312). This is the concern of a lover and registers differently than the quasi-clinical (albeit affectionate) observations of Molly. For the lover, illness provides the perfect cover for openly talking about the object of one's affection: "Molly, how ill your sister is looking! What is it? Has she had advice? You must forgive me, but so often those who live together in the same house don't observe the first approaches of illness" (312). Here, Roger puts his scientific training to medical use, reasoning that one must step back and take in the whole picture to see the story's evolution over time, to compare the past with the present condition to recognize change. Roger's concern shows not only how attuned he is to Cynthia's appearance of health but also how far he is willing to go to express his feelings—he has, in effect, accused the town doctor of failing to do his job. Of whom would Cynthia receive expert "advice" but her stepfather, the doctor? To be sure, we have already seen that Mr. Gibson has difficulty recognizing that his own daughter has grown, but when it comes to symptoms of illness, he has yet to fail. Roger's questions masquerade as objective concern for medical neglect, and he begins to offer his own advice, advice that would allow him to see Cynthia more regularly: "I wonder if she wants a change of air? . . . I do wish we could have her at Hamley Hall" (312).

That Roger engages Molly under the auspices of a kind of professional concern helps to hand the authority over Cynthia's case to Molly. Rather than approaching the doctor with these remedies, he defers to Molly, asking if there is "anything [he] can do for [her] sister." He says, "We have plenty of books . . . Or flowers? she likes flowers. Oh! And our forced strawberries are just ready—I will bring some to-morrow" (313). Roger uses Cynthia's "indisposition" as an excuse for visiting almost every day, bringing "some fresh offering" (313). This affection, which Molly knows is not reciprocated, keeps her on the outside, as an observer instead of the preventionist she would rather be: "I must wait and watch, and see if I can do anything for [Roger]" (354). By presenting Molly as a long-suffering unacknowledged lover who, like Austen's Fanny Price, "did not know her own feelings," Gaskell allows her heroine to identify her role in clearer terms than we see with Fanny (354). She realizes that although it is beyond her power to prevent Roger from falling in love, she might in observing his symptoms closely be all the better positioned to administer proper treatment to his broken heart when the occasion arises. Molly can foretell Roger's pain because she has observed enough of Cynthia's heart (without knowing the particulars of her situation) to know that her affections are "out of [his] reach" (354).

Molly has, by now, become an educated observer, and Gaskell is clear to distinguish hers from other types of examinations that go on in the novel. Her interest in Cynthia is one of "affection" rather than "the coarser desire of knowing everything for a little excitement." It is linked more with Roger's interest in natural science and her father's attention to his patients than with the social cares of her mother or the other women of Hollingford. She sees and hears everything not to gratify her curiosity but to know what to do and how to act. Molly "cho[oses] to use" only "delicate instruments" to break through the "dead wall[s]" Cynthia builds (414). Certainly, a more curious heroine would have extracted the truth from Cynthia much sooner. We witness Molly's delicacy or naïveté at the ball, where she suspects that Mr. Preston has some "power over" Cynthia but cannot determine what it is. She does not have the data (nor do we) to figure out that Mr. Preston has blackmailed Cynthia into marriage. Indeed, even the women most schooled in these matters do not suspect such a plight. The difference is that Molly is surprised when she finds out about Cynthia's liaison, while someone like Lady Harriet suspects all along that Cynthia "is the real heroine of this story" (526).

When Molly finally learns about Cynthia and Preston's secret engagement, she approaches it with literal as well as social medicine, for although Cynthia works herself into a physical frenzy, requiring some medical attention, she primarily needs a moral intervention. Molly stumbles upon the couple arguing in the bushes and, finding Cynthia "hysterical" and unable to move, takes it upon herself to "restore [Cynthia's] calmness" (461). She orders Preston to get water from a cottage nearby, which temporarily gets rid of him but eventually becomes part of the evidence used to sully Molly's name. Molly's job, as she sees it, is to help "extricate Cynthia . . .

by thought, or advice, or action" from what has become a dangerous and physically traumatic entanglement (464). While Molly's desire to protect Roger, who has by now professed his love to Cynthia, motivates her, we also know that she would have acted on Cynthia's behalf without considering his interest. Molly's energies seem focused almost entirely on diagnosing and treating Cynthia, which delays Molly's own marriage plot but allows her to represent the value of telling one's own story and the importance of a competent listener.

Anticipating the kind of therapy that Sigmund Freud would develop at the beginning of the following century, Gaskell presents Cynthia's confession to Molly as a talking cure. Although Cynthia's story is a secret rather than a repressed memory or emotion, Gaskell moves us from somatic medicine and the physical exam of the father to the psychological and narrative medicine of the daughter. If we had not yet seen the parallels between Molly's actions and her father's profession, we do now. Mr. Gibson offered a similar treatment to Cynthia during the first signs of her "indisposition," but for him, the talk was not itself the remedy. What Cynthia refused the father, she willingly gives to his daughter, and Molly determines the course to be taken: "Lie down on the bed, and I will sit by you, and let us talk it over. . . . When did it all begin?" Cynthia refuses to lie down but agrees, with Molly's prompting, to speak. The story functions as both a case history and a form of cure. Cynthia finally gets to tell a story that is more about a mother's neglect than about the imminent problem of a coerced engagement. As if we are back in that fairy-tale opening of "Once upon a time," Cynthia begins her story: "Long ago—four or five years. I was such a child to be left all to myself" (467). A story that begins with children left alone cannot end well. We learn that Hyacinth left Cynthia alone during a holiday when the latter was slightly younger than Molly is now, and although she gave Cynthia permission to visit another family, she did not give her any money for the journey. Mr. Preston filled the void left by the mother, offering sympathy and money. Eventually, when it came to pass that Cynthia could not repay the debt, Mr.

Preston extracted a promise of marriage, which was to be repaid when Cynthia turned twenty. That time is now, and the payment is due. Mr. Preston has threatened to show the letters in which Cynthia dilates on her mother's many faults. As much as Cynthia disdains her mother, she does not want her mother's faults to face public scrutiny. More specifically, she does not want Mr. Gibson to read the letters. As Cynthia begins to tell her story, Molly notices that "an aged and careworn expression . . . had taken temporary hold of the brilliant and beautiful face" (467). But once she reveals her story and Molly determines the remedy, Cynthia, crying "out of weariness and despair of mind," nonetheless regains her former countenance, as she "presse[s] the beautiful head to [Molly's] bosom" (474).

Molly's subsequent actions on behalf of Cynthia recast Molly as the heroine of a dangerous seduction plot, something her father attempted to prevent when he sent her to Hamley. But unlike Cynthia, she knowingly and with purpose puts herself—as a doctor might—in harm's way to bring this portion of the story to a close, in order to comfort and prevent further harm. When she confronts Mr. Preston, Molly sounds strikingly like her father when he reasoned with Mr. Coxe about the inappropriateness of his affection for Molly. When Preston claims that Cynthia gave her promise to marry him "as solemnly as ever woman—," Molly cuts him off before he can finish, asserting (quite rightly) that "[s]he was not a woman, she was only a girl, barely sixteen" (480). Unlike her father, Molly has got it right—she sees the sex and power disparity represented in her young age. The illness from which Cynthia suffers is much less physical than social and moral, but it still demands medicalized (if not specifically medical) treatment and has everything to do with the power of narrative. Molly retrieves the written documents and redirects Cynthia's plot toward its closure.

What acts as closure for Cynthia, who represents the crisis-cure model of narrative action, threatens to place Molly within a similar trajectory. The town speculates about Molly's propriety, which turns her into the focus of diagnostic scrutiny. Gaskell imagines the fallout from Cynthia's plot as a sanitationist might, for Molly is temporarily "defiled" because of her contact with Cynthia's story. The tête-à-tête with Preston and the presumed privacy of such an interaction can mean only one thing when witnessed in public: that the two are engaged in some secretive, potentially sexual liaison. When Mr. Gibson learns that his daughter has been "carrying on a clandestine correspondence with Mr. Preston" (513)—the very activity he prevented Molly from participating in with Mr. Coxe—he warns her that the "slight[est] thing may blacken a girl's reputation for life" (518) and accuses Cynthia of "dragging Molly's name down into the same mire" (543). Mr. Gibson moves between the language of sanitation and theories of contagion, first imagining Molly's situation in terms of filth but then crediting Cynthia with transmitting it. Rather than handing over the case to Mr. Gibson, however, Gaskell uses Molly's condition to bolster the daughter's authority.

Once the "reports" of Molly's behavior with Mr. Preston "are abroad," she is treated as a public threat, and the town fixates on her as the dangerous contaminant: "Mrs. Goodenough openly pull[s] her grand-daughter away" from Molly (507). When Mr. Gibson learns of this kind of treatment, he wishes he "had the doctoring of these slanderous gossips" so that he can "make their tongues lie still for a while" (513). Molly rejects her father's brand of treatment, invoking a maintenance model instead of therapeutics. She refuses to allow him to engage in any sinister act, even if only in his thoughts, explaining to him that the situation must run its course, that he must be "patient with the gossip and cackle" (519). While she correctly assumes that her father's remedy would not cure, she does not quite realize that something must be done. The only way to prove Molly's innocence and to prevent serious harm is to demonstrate that contact with her is not only safe but also desirable. Lady Harriet, a woman who has always been drawn to Molly's morality and knows a bit about how stories can heal, spends the day in total contact with Molly. Her social rank has the power to prove, with one handshake,

Molly's innocence more than any "doctoring" Mr. Gibson could do. She walks Molly through town and finally "stand[s] on the white door-steps, at the Miss Brownings', . . . holding Molly's hand while she wish[s] her good-by" (533). Molly, who does not realize all that Lady Harriet has done for her, is no longer a blight; she stands as an emblem of purity in that transitional space between the street and the home. Though Lady Harriet takes control over Molly's treatment, Molly herself knows to take her case out of her father's hands.

Molly has successfully escaped contamination and maintained Cynthia's health, but these are social rather than physical problems. And although the language of medicine permeates these episodes, it is not until Molly takes part in Osborne Hamley's treatment that we see her engage more directly with the practice of medicine. Though she has a deep affection for the entire Hamley family, her relationship to Osborne is the least intimate and most disinterested. She is objective without losing her sympathetic care. Her final case, one that will lead to her own physical illness, pits doctor against daughter in a decidedly professional encounter. When word comes to the Gibsons that Osborne Hamley is dead, the doctor is out and Molly determines to go in his place. To the repeated question "Is the doctor coming, Miss?" Molly decides, "I will go myself" (550). As if recalling the Squire's earlier claim that having the doctor's daughter is "nearly as good as the doctor," she does not hesitate to think that she will be a satisfactory substitute, at least in this case, when the patient is already dead. And indeed she is. Molly finds the Squire in serious distress and convinces him to take a spoonful of soup. The Squire even requests that Molly stay the night, and Mr. Gibson, unsure whether it is the right thing to do, allows Molly to decide. She agrees, and Molly and her father engage in a postmortem of Osborne's case:

> "[W]hat did Osborne die of?" She asked the question in a low awe-stricken voice.
>
> "Something wrong with the heart. You wouldn't understand if I told you. I apprehended it for some time; but

> it is better not to talk of such things at home. When I saw him on Thursday week, he seemed better than I have seen him for a long time. I told Dr. Nicholls so. But one never can calculate in these complaints."
>
> "You saw him Thursday week? Why, you never mentioned it!" said Molly. (554)

Mr. Gibson responds abruptly: "No. I don't talk of my patients at home. Besides, I didn't want him to consider me as his doctor, but as a friend. Any alarm about his own health would only have hastened the catastrophe." This exchange begins simply enough—as a discussion between a layperson and an authority, a daughter and her doctor-father. Molly is "awe-stricken" by the gravity of her own question, but it is her interest in the cause of death that marks her as something more than a grieving friend or family member—the Squire never asks what killed Osborne. And while her father asserts his authority and her relative ignorance ("You wouldn't understand"), he does share the details of Osborne's treatment, explaining what he knew, when he knew it, and with whom he consulted. The doctor asserts a protective division between "home" and work that has already been tested by his wife by making a distinction between the personal and the professional—a doctor, it seems, can only demonstrate friendship by *not* talking about health.

But Molly pursues the point, because something in her father's response does not quite fit her experience with the case. She probes the point about Osborne's own knowledge:

> "Then he didn't know that he was ill—ill of a dangerous complaint, I mean: one that might end as it has done?"
>
> "No; certainly not. He would only have been watching his symptoms—accelerating matters, in fact."
>
> "Oh! papa!" said Molly, shocked.
>
> "I've no time to go into the question," Mr. Gibson continued. "And until you know what has to be said on both sides, and in every instance, you are not qualified to judge." (554)

The authority shifts when Molly challenges her father's decision to withhold information from Osborne. Mr. Gibson interprets her "shock" as an accusation—Osborne should have been told—and feels compelled to defend his actions by reminding her that she is not "qualified to judge" his decision. If we think back to Mrs. Gibson's "diagnosis" of Osborne's future, we recall a similar reflex on the part of the doctor. In that instance, Mrs. Gibson was correct in what she overheard, though the use to which she put the information was faulty and ineffective. In this case, Molly is correct in thinking that her father was wrong for withholding information and for thinking that Osborne was unaware of his health. And because the novel has been working toward developing her judgment, Molly's response displays a level of knowledge worth attending to. Both Mrs. Gibson and Molly intrude on the doctor's territory, but with different results.

Gaskell highlights this contest between father and daughter structurally, by transferring Osborne's case over to Molly in the next chapter. Chapter 51 ends with Mr. Gibson telling Molly to go to bed, and chapter 52 continues the scene but begins with Molly's revelation of Osborne's secret: "Papa, I think I ought to tell you something. I know a great secret of Osborne's, which I promised not to tell; but the last time I saw him I think he must have been afraid of something like this" (555). This scene is the only instance in which Gaskell places a chapter break in the middle of a conversation, as if to divide Molly's authority from her father's. To be sure, Molly begins sobbing as she shares this information, but, realizing her moral and—we might say—professional responsibility, she "suddenly master[s] herself" and continues. In telling her father about Osborne's secret marriage and child, Molly speculates that, contrary to her father's belief in his patient's ignorance, Osborne knew he was dying. She recalls for her father the day when Osborne came to their house "to see [Mr. Gibson] professionally" (492). The doctor was away, but as she had done with Cynthia's case, Molly took over for her father and gave Osborne the chance and the time to talk. Molly controlled the session by telling Osborne not to "go on talking so fast." She advised him, "Rest. No one will interrupt us" (493–94), recognizing that talking would alleviate his anxiety. Although no cure, talking was the only palliative that would do any good at the time. Osborne claimed, "I feel better already now I feel that some one else knows the whereabouts of my wife and child" (494). Molly listened to Osborne then and retells the story to her father now, actions that, though they do not save the patient, pave the way for his son, the Hamley heir, to heal the ailing estate.

DOCTORED DAUGHTER

At the height of Molly's medical assertiveness, Gaskell pulls her out of the role as the doctoring daughter and turns her into her father's patient. The desire to sustain health in the midst of so much disease and dis-ease, which has thus far generated this narrative, yields to sickness and to a traditional plot of crisis and recovery. Once Osborne's wife and son appear on the scene, Molly becomes sick with grief and in the early stages of scarlet fever, her body breaking down, unable to sustain the constant mental and physical labor. She waits until after she hears that Osborne's widow is on the mend before admitting to her father that she feels "unaccountably weary" (580). Molly begins to describe her symptoms, thus transforming from a consulting partner to a patient. Her father responds swiftly and authoritatively, blaming himself for failing to notice earlier and for giving her too much responsibility. He does not diagnose her with any disease, saying only that "[s]he has been overworked, and I've been a fool" (582). When he gets Molly home, Mr. Gibson's concern that her "illness might be a precursor of a still worse malady" comes to pass. Although not "acute," her case is severe enough to make him "fea[r] that she might become a permanent invalid" (583). As Molly's apprenticeship ends, her romance begins. No longer does she listen to or tell stories that heal others. And yet, even by ending with Molly in her invalid gown, the narrative of health remains a persistent force—we are not reminded of Mrs. Hamley or the first Mrs. Gibson, nor do we see Molly quite within the tradition of crisis needing cure. For although her body has been (must be) inured by sickness so that she may regain her position as the novel's center and narrative focus, we are left with the promise of a future wife who has the authority of both a mother and a doctor.

Confined once more to her bed, Molly appears as a body in need of a cure. Mr. Gibson associates "nervous fever" with her recent overwork, but this is not the first time she has been ill. The narrator first mentions concern over Molly's health well before her encounter with Mr. Preston. Shortly after her father's marriage and Roger's proposal to Cynthia, the narrator explains that "she . . . gradually [fell] into low health, rather than bad health. Her heart beat more feebly and slower" (411). The thought that her father knows his wife's faults but cannot fix them—and that Roger fails to see Cynthia's faults—seems to cause a "languor . . . [and] slow depression of manner" (420). In this regard, Molly first seems a rather typical "heroine"; her breaking heart (both filial or romantic) leads to physical illness, or at least to the kind of delicacy associated with young women in love. But Gaskell does not take us down this road; Molly's illnesses function much more ambiguously, in part because Gaskell has been training her all along to become a practitioner of domestic medicine. The next time we hear of Molly's "delicate health," the narrator attributes it to "rapid growth during the last few months" (446). Molly is not, then, the sickly heroine waiting for a curative encounter with her beloved; she is, rather, a growing girl, experiencing the physical pain that comes with a physiological reality. The idea that Molly's body seems to be growing too fast has metaphorical resonances; she can physically, not just mentally, feel the effects of becoming a woman.

Curiously, Molly's illnesses do not build over the course of the novel toward the eventual invalidism that gets her father's notice. Rather, we can read her "low health" and "growing pains" as separate incidents attributed to different causes. By the time Molly becomes an invalid at the end of the novel, she has been introduced into the tradition of lovesick women. And while her earlier lapses bespeak a delicate constitution, Gaskell is careful to distinguish these moments from the kind of physical and mental labor that leads to Molly's fever—as her father says, "She has been overworked." Indeed, she has been. While with the Hamleys, she has to care for the Squire, who becomes frighteningly insensible: when she first attempts to soothe him, he suddenly cries out, "thr[owing] himself across the corpse, and we[eping] in such a terrible manner that Molly trem[bles] lest he should die" (553). After the arrival of Osborne's secret wife, Aimee Osborne, and her son, Molly must look out for the interests of the grieving and ailing widow. When the Squire begins to complain to Mr. Gibson about Osborne's refusal to tell him about the wife, "Molly gr[ows] impatient on the mother's behalf," telling her father that "[Aimee] [i]s very ill; perhaps worse than we think" (577). She asserts her diagnostic authority, because she knows something about the toll of clandestine love affairs. Her turn to sickness forces us to recall what the narrative has been asking her to know and learn about the powerful relationship between medicine, management, and narrative.

Overwork may be the initial cause of her illness, but its effect is that she becomes the primary object of desire and experiences the benefits of her own medical treatment: released from the professional plot of sustained health, she gets to tell her own sad tale. Mr. Gibson initially prescribes "a trashy novel or two" to help Molly sleep, but it is by rehearsing the story of Osborne's death and his wife's sudden arrival to Cynthia that "Molly's health and spirits improv[e] rapidly" (586). Cynthia allows Molly to "continually recu[r] to all the time of distress and sorrow at Hamley Hall," because, as the narrator explains, Cynthia "instinctively knew that the repetition of all these painful recollections would ease the oppressed memory, which refused to dwell on anything but what had occurred at a time of feverish disturbance of health." Mrs. Gibson, by contrast, only says, "You told me that before, my dear. Let's talk of something else" (586). Thus, by the time Roger sees Molly in her "pretty white invalid's dress" (592), she has recovered just enough to become, as he observes, "the delicate fragrant beauty" of his brother's prediction (593).

Illness not only reunites Molly with Roger but also removes Cynthia from the picture and makes way for the suspended romance plot. After Molly recovers from her more serious nervous fever, she contracts a rather convenient and harmless cold that keeps her and the reader away from Cynthia's wedding. For with Mr. Preston out of the way, Cynthia is free to marry Mr. Henderson. We are relocated to Cumnor Towers, where Molly's love plot speeds toward the inevitable conclusion. With Roger as a guest at the Towers, the stage is set for the convalescing heroine to find comfort from a newly professed lover. But instead of allowing for sickroom confessionals or care to bring Roger and Molly together, Gaskell returns to a model of prevention—quarantine—that, ironically, becomes the obstacle keeping them apart. Once again, Molly's plot is framed as medical intervention. Scarlet fever, which helped bring Roger and Molly together earlier in the novel, now keeps them separated. Recall that Molly's extended stay at Hamley in the beginning of the novel was the result of her governess (Miss Eyre) being in contact with her nephew who suffered from scarlet fever. Now, Osborne's child contracts scarlet fever, the "one illness [Mr. Gibson] dread[s]" (639), because Molly has no immunity against it; "from the strict quarantine her father evidently thought it necessary to establish between the two houses, she was not likely to see Roger again before his departure for Africa" (640).

The closest we come to a marriage proposal occurs during a discussion between Roger and Mr. Gibson, which turns into a medical encounter. When Roger reveals his disappointment in not being able to see Molly again before he leaves, Mr. Gibson "turn[s] his keen, observant eyes upon the young man, and look[s] at him in as penetrating a manner as if he had been beginning some unknown illness" (641). And of course, to some degree it is a type of illness.

Once Roger pours out his feelings to "the doctor and the father" (641), Mr. Gibson acknowledges that he would "rather give [his] child . . . to [Roger] than to any other man in the world!" (643). This does not change the medical risks involved if the lovers were to meet. Once again, Mr. Gibson asserts his professional and paternal authority, denying Roger's request to see Molly with a resounding "Decidedly not. There I come in as a doctor as well as a father. No!" (644). The doctor-father regains control of the narrative by calling on the logic of prevention and asserting yet another prescription. This time, though, it is no joke. Mr. Gibson is on firm professional and domestic ground. The doctor returns Molly to quarantine with reasons based on sound preventative medicine. It is a true quarantine, for the lovers know why they will be separated, and through the sequestration, Gaskell creates the kind delay that serves to heighten our anticipation for their union and for the narrative's closure. With poor Mr. Coxe, Molly never knew she was separated from a possible romance—the one-sided quarantine served not to provide closure so much as to offer the opportunity for other forms of contact to initiate narrative. For Molly and Roger—and for the novel more generally—the separation and the tension that the more recent quarantine creates keeps everyone healthy and keeps the story alive. It provides an ending without foreclosing the novel too abruptly—an openness that is underlined by the unfinished state of the novel.

Had Gaskell lived long enough to complete the final number, she would have, the *Cornhill* editor tells us, "charmingly . . . drawn" Roger and Molly's reunion. Instead, we get an ending—a better ending, perhaps—that reminds us of where we have seen Molly before. We find her again looking out a window onto a day that she "was afraid would never never come" (6). But this Molly has learned to modulate her emotions and to manage her health. Instead of an overexcited little girl who makes herself sick or an innocent young woman whose father must secretly manage her affairs, she is "happy, glowing, sad, and content" (645). The "sadness," here, speaks to her separation from Roger, the risk involved in his journey to Africa, and the inability to finally speak of her love (it is still merely "friendship" [645]). It also reflects the combined authority and perspective she has gained from being a doctoring (and now doctored) daughter. For even though Molly does not become quite the expert that modern readers might hope she will become—she does not seem destined to write any medical tracts—she nevertheless brings us closer to a model of medical practice that requires narrative competence. Gaskell did not intend to conclude *Wives and Daughters* with Molly's ambivalence—the editor explains that Molly was to be "happier than" Roger (649)—but it is a more fitting ending to a novel that has throughout been preoccupied, as was the culture in which it was produced, with the never-ending work that goes into preserving health and the ever-ongoing difficulty of managing stories.

Afterword

Health in Narrative Medicine

I begin this book by citing John Ruskin's complaint about the illicit scenarios and vile characters featured in certain Victorian novels. While it may or may not agree with Ruskin's evaluation of Dickens and Eliot, recent scholarship has nonetheless affirmed and fruitfully accounted for the ubiquity of literal and metaphorical sickness in fiction. This book, although not denying the significance of disease in the Victorian novel, focuses on fictional and medical perspectives on health, seeking to articulate the components—the narrative structures and imperatives—that define them. As each of the chapters demonstrates, medical advice by professionals and nonprofessionals of the Victorian era was, perhaps like Ruskin's literary advice, concerned that readers were often too fixated on illness. These "therapeutic" reading practices—ones that center on treatments and cures—tend to obscure "hygienic" modes of reading, ones that are defined primarily by prevention and maintenance. The novel stages, through its content and form, this tension between the seductiveness associated with the often-melodramatic crisis and recovery and the banality of prophylaxis and routine. Thus, while the writers featured in this book—and the plots, characters, and metaphors they drew on for social critique—often relied, as critics have demonstrated, on literal and figurative disease, they were equally invested in preventative plots, in transforming contagion and contagious characters into salubrious contact and imagining physical wellness as central to the authority of the autobiographical "I," while recognizing that omniscient narration's healthy perspective governs and is itself governed by the "peculiar privileges" of invalidism, and in mining the psychological as well as somatic health that ensues when narrative and medical competence are equally involved.

The texts I examine in this book—from late eighteenth-century domestic medical manuals to mid-Victorian novels and public health reports—attempt to teach their readers not only what health is (to the extent that that is possible) but also how to read for it, distorting the divide between doctor and patient. When reading medical advice about health (rather than disease), one is both a patient and a practitioner, imagining the treatment and consequences of future disease as a means of avoiding it. Keeping in good health is anything but easy, and sometimes it proves impossible; the difficulty of this task—of maintaining and telling one's health narrative—requires constant attention, impinging as it does on multiple aspects of one's story. For the Victorian novelist, issues of middle-class domesticity and marriage, individual identity, social theory and reform, and professional ethics determined the role that health would play in their novels, just as the desire to know health shaped their novelistic treatment of these topics.

The first two parts of this book are concerned with separating therapeutics from hygiene, emphasizing the latter, first to draw out health's narrative and social value, and second to demonstrate what "hygienic" reading might involve. The third part's focus on *Wives and Daughters* offers a more panoramic view, drawing together therapeutics and hygiene as well as somatic and psychological ailments and placing them on equal ground. As Galen puts it, while we may (and need to) recognize that there are two "subdivisions" of medicine, the "path of investigation for both is the same."[1] And as we can see in Gaskell's novel, the best practitioners of this "science" are good storytellers and listeners; they are proficient in both narrative modes (hygiene and therapeutics) and in the ways these narratives overlap and inform one another. I want to conclude my study of nineteenth-century novels and medical narratives by jumping ahead in time to illuminate the degree to which the narrative competence and ethical reading practices these novels invite shape contemporary professional practice, particularly current medical education.

Reading for Health is concerned, sometimes implicitly and sometimes explicitly, with the question of narrative competence (a phrase that I apply to Molly Gibson's proficiency), particularly the doctor's (in)ability to talk to and about his patients. For noted narratologist Gerald Prince, "narrative competence" is the internalization of the "set of rules and intuitions . . . that allow readers to produce and process narratives."[2] We readers, whether we can articulate these "rules" (of health, of narrative) or not, possess the competence to understand them and to create narratives of our own. In a 2001 article in *JAMA: The Journal of the American Medical Association*, Rita Charon applies this concept to medical practice, suggesting, "The effective practice of medicine requires narrative competence, that is, the ability to acknowledge, absorb, interpret, and act on the stories and plights of others."[3] She calls this type of practice "narrative medicine," and for Charon and others, the narrative competence that distinguishes it from more traditional approaches to the clinical encounter and to medical education is part of a larger ethics of reading, as it "enables the physician to practice medicine with empathy, reflection, professionalism, and trustworthiness."[4]

Although the relationship between medicine and narrative, between stories and medical care, is not new, the field of study called "narrative medicine" is, and its role in medical education has become increasingly important.[5] Several institutions in and outside of the United States offer lectures and workshops as well as courses and degrees in narrative medicine.[6] In the course I team-teach at the University of Southern California's Keck School of Medicine, for example, students read fiction, poetry, and theory, and they write personal and patient narratives to become more attentive to the nuanced ways that stories unfold and to understand how we make sense of any given narrative. They practice close reading, using terms and concepts from literary analysis—point of view, metaphor, repetition, silence, shifts in temporality—to identify how the various features of a narrative shape the teller's sense of self and how such tactics reveal what the teller needs from her listener and what patients and their physicians need from each other to engage in a more compassionate and, as we tell our students, more efficient form of medicine.[7]

The work in narrative medicine understandably emphasizes illness and death, considering what it means to be a healer, particularly when cure is not possible or when cure is not enough. Illness is a time when the individual is most vulnerable, when, as Shlomith Rimmon-Kenan and Arthur Frank have argued,[8] the narrative that personally defines the subject gets disrupted, perhaps irrevocably so, and a new narrative takes over, one motivated by the promise of recovery or the fear of death, or suspended in a state (the chaos) of uncertainty. Although my intention is not to challenge such a focus, *Reading for Health* invites interpretative methods that are more attuned to the narratives of health, to the ways that prevention and maintenance, patience and routine enter into the narratives that define who we are and what we "weak mortals" do as doctors and patients, literary scholars and students, writers and readers.

Notes

INTRODUCTION

Chapter epigraphs: John Ruskin, "Fiction, Fair and Foul," in *The Works of John Ruskin*, ed. E. T. Cook and Alexander Wedderburn (London: Longmans, Green, 1908), 274; Alexander I. Shand, "The Pleasures of Sickness," *Blackwood's Edinburgh Magazine* 145 (April 1889): 546.

1. Although it does not focus on the Victorian novel, Susan Sontag's *Illness as Metaphor* (New York: Vintage Books, 1979) is one of the earliest studies to explore the link between disease and art, particularly the metaphors surrounding tuberculosis and cancer. In addition to Miriam Bailin's seminal work, *The Sickroom in Victorian Fiction: The Art of Being Ill* (Cambridge: Cambridge University Press, 1995), see Athena Vrettos, *Somatic Fictions: Imagining Illness in Victorian Culture* (Stanford: Stanford University Press, 1995); Pamela K. Gilbert, *Disease, Desire, and the Body in Victorian Women's Popular Novels* (Cambridge: Cambridge University Press, 1997); Catherine Judd, *Bedside Seductions: Nursing and the Victorian Imagination, 1830–1880* (New York: St. Martin's Press, 1998); Erin O'Connor, *Raw Material: Producing Pathology in Victorian Culture* (Durham, NC: Duke University Press, 2000); Jane Wood, *Passion and Pathology in Victorian Fiction* (Oxford: Oxford University Press, 2001); Martha Stoddard Holmes, *Fictions of Affliction: Physical Disability in Victorian Culture* (Ann Arbor: University of Michigan Press, 2004); and Maria Frawley, *Invalidism and Identity in Nineteenth-Century Britain* (Chicago: University of Chicago Press, 2004). For American literature, see Diane Price Herndl, *Invalid Women: Figuring Feminine Illness in American Fiction and Culture, 1840–1940* (Chapel Hill: University of North Carolina Press, 1993); and Cynthia Davis, *Bodily and Narrative Forms: The Influence of Medicine on American Literature, 1845–1915* (Stanford: Stanford University Press, 2000).

2. Bailin, *Sickroom in Victorian Fiction*, 5.

3. Ruskin conceded, "There is some excuse . . . for the pathologic labour of the modern novelist in the fact that he cannot easily, in a city population, find a healthy mind to vivisect" (*Works of John Ruskin*, 281).

4. The editors of the 1908 edition of "Fiction, Fair and Foul" note that Ruskin's theory about Scott—that his "perfect novels were written in unclouded days and

before physical suffering"—does not hold up entirely. They explain, "*Rob Roy* is included by Ruskin in his theories of the perfect and untainted novels; and yet, as Lockhart relates, *Rob Roy* was written in acute pain." E. T. Cook and Alexander Wedderburn, introduction to *The Works of John Ruskin* (London: Longmans, Green, 1908), xxxiv.

5. Bruce Haley, *The Healthy Body and Victorian Culture* (Cambridge, MA: Harvard University Press, 1978), 46.

6. Carlyle quoted in ibid., 46. Haley makes the point that "that sort of clinical vocabulary strikes us as crude and unpalatable" (46).

7. Walter Bagehot, "The Waverley Novels," in *The Collected Works of Walter Bagehot*, ed. Norman St. John–Stevas (Cambridge, MA: Harvard University Press, 1965), 56.

8. Although critics address the ways in which an author's experience with illness affects her work, they tend not to judge a work's aesthetic successes or failures based on these biographical details. See Bailin, *Sickroom in Victorian Fiction*, especially her discussion of Charlotte Brontë. A notable exception to this critical attention would be D. A. Miller, *Jane Austen, or the Secret of Style* (Princeton: Princeton University Press, 2003). For Miller, *Sanditon*, the novel Austen died before finishing, marks the "breakdown . . . of Austen Style" (80), as if illness caused Austen to lose control of her language and thus, finally, reveal herself in her prose.

9. Kirstie Blair, "Pathologizing the Victorians," *Interdisciplinary Literary Studies: A Journal of Criticism and Theory* 3, no. 2 (2002): 138.

10. Roger Cooter, "The Traffic in Victorian Bodies: Medicine, Literature, and History," *Victorian Studies: An Interdisciplinary Journal of Social, Political, and Cultural Studies* 45, no. 3 (2003): 516.

11. There are exceptions to this generalization. Martin Wallen's *City of Health, Fields of Disease: Revolutions in the Poetry, Medicine, and Philosophy of Romanticism* (Aldershot, UK: Ashgate, 2004) and Pamela Gilbert's *The Citizen's Body: Desire, Health, and the Social in Victorian England* (Columbus: Ohio State University Press, 2007), for example, focus critical attention on health. Wallen examines how poetry, medicine, and philosophy define and articulate the opposition between health and disease. Gilbert demonstrates how Victorian conceptions of fitness became central to the construction of individual and social identity and thus to the creation of the English citizen in a liberal society. For an intriguing discussion of life insurance designations of "healthy enough," see Timothy Alborn's "Normal Bodies, Normal Prices in Victorian Life Insurance," *RaVon* 49 (February 2008): [online, 42 paragraphs].

12. Important recent work that examines the disease experience includes, for example, Jason Daniel Tougow's *Strange Cases: The Medical Case History and the British Novel* (New York: Routledge, 2006) and Meegan Kennedy's *Revising the Clinic: Vision and Representations in Victorian Medical Narratives*

and the Novel (Columbus: Ohio State University Press, 2010), which both focus on case studies. Susan Zeiger's *Inventing the Addict: Drugs, Race, and Sexuality in Nineteenth-Century British and American Literature* (Amherst: University of Massachusetts Press, 2008) broadens the discussion of pathology to include drug addiction.

13. While my thinking on health has been shaped by Michel Foucault's work on medical professionals and institutions, particularly his examination of the space of the clinic and his view of the changing role of the patient, my work does not explicitly invoke a Foucauldian methodology or history. In *Literature and Medicine in Nineteenth-Century Britain: From Mary Shelley to George Eliot* (Cambridge: Cambridge University Press, 2008), Janis McLarren Caldwell cautions against "map[ping] Foucault's reading of French history onto the British scene" (6), while Kennedy's *Revising the Clinic* makes the point that not all doctors adopt a Foucauldian gaze. Medical historian Dora B. Weiner's *Citizen-Patient in Revolutionary and Imperial Paris* (Baltimore, MD: Johns Hopkins University Press, 1993) acknowledges the importance of Foucault's work but suggests that when we move outside of Foucault's archive another version of the doctor and the clinic emerges. These works have opened space for my study, which I see as offering a perspective on health—a way of reading for it—in the nineteenth century that is adjacent rather than opposed to Foucault's approach.

14. See also Roy Porter and Dorothy Porter's *In Sickness and in Health: The British Experience, 1650–1850* (New York: Blackwell, 1988) and Andrew Wear's *Medicine in Society: Historical Essays* (Cambridge: Cambridge University Press, 1992).

15. Vrettos, *Somatic Fictions*, 2.

16. John Wiltshire, *Jane Austen and the Body: "The Picture of Health"* (Cambridge: Cambridge University Press, 1992), 9.

17. Robert James, *A Medicinal Dictionary*, 3 vols. (London: Printed for T. Osborne, 1743–45), lxvi.

18. Miller, *Jane Austen*, ix (emphasis added).

19. John Sinclair, *The Code of Health and Longevity*, 4th ed. (London: B. McMillan, 1818), 12.

20. Thomas Beddoes, *Manual of Health; or, Conducting the Invalid Safely through the Seasons* (London: Johnson, 1806), 7.

21. James Hinton, *Thoughts on Health and Some of Its Conditions* (London: Smith, Elder, 1871), 3.

22. The assumption that people ignore health (whether this is true or not) has circulated since the days of ancient medicine. Galen, one of the most prolific medical writers of his time, was particularly critical of athletes for ignoring prevailing advice about health: "Athletics," he claims "is the cultivation, not of health, but of disease." See *Galen: Selected Works*, ed. P. N. Singer, Oxford World's Classics Series (Oxford: Oxford University Press, 1997), 48. Such warnings are

both an assessment of a cultural attitude toward health and an effective rhetorical strategy for claiming authority and making one's advice essential.

23. John Milner Fothergill, *The Maintenance of Health: A Medical Work for Lay Readers* (London: Smith, Elder, 1874).

24. Galen, *Hygiene (De sanitate tuenda)*, trans. Robert Montraville Green (Springfield, IL: Charles C. Thomas, 1951), 5.

25. P. N. Singer, introduction to *Galen: Selected Works*, Oxford World's Classics Series (Oxford: Oxford University Press, 1997), xix.

26. *Galen: Selected Works*, 5.

27. William Strange, *The Restoration of Health; or, The Application of the Laws of Hygiene to the Recovery of Health, Forming a Manual for the Invalid and a Guide in the Sick-Room* (London: Longmans, Green, 1865). The typically unwieldy full title of his text reflects its therapeutic focus. His work from the year before, *Seven Sources of Health* (London: Henry Renshaw, 1864) focuses on prevention more than recovery.

28. My understanding of eighteenth- and nineteenth-century readers' responses to medical practice and beliefs about their bodies has been shaped by Bruce Haley's suggestive claims about Victorian definitions of health, as well as by the invaluable studies of cultural and political attitudes about health by medical historians such as Roy Porter and Dorothy Porter.

29. I focus on novelistic fiction because the aims and scope of novels and medical advice are of a piece. I also find justification for my focus on novels in Sir John Sinclair's claim in *The Code of Health and Longevity*, vol. 3 (Edinburgh: Arch Constable, 1807) that although there have been useful poems on the subject, it is "dangerous . . . to prescribe rules in verse, on such a delicate subject as health, because the muse may occasionally elevate the poet above the reach of salutary precepts, and make him forget the *physician*" (4). He cites as exempt from this general rule "Regimen Santitatis Salerni," composed in 1099 by Johannes de Mediolanus.

30. Peter Brooks, *Reading for the Plot: Design and Intention in Narrative* (Cambridge, MA: Harvard University Press, 1984); D. A. Miller, *Narrative and Its Discontents: Problems of Closure in the Traditional Novel* (Princeton: Princeton University Press, 1989).

31. Brooks, *Reading for the Plot*, 47, 53 (original emphasis). In *The Sense of an Ending: Studies in the Theory of Fiction* (Oxford: Oxford University Press, 1966), Frank Kermode sees this desire in terms of apocalyptic thinking.

32. Brooks, *Reading for the Plot*, 138 (emphasis added), 139.

33. Miller, *Narrative and Its Discontents*, ix.

34. Ibid., 27, xiv, 20.

35. See also D. A. Miller, "The Late Jane Austen," *Raritan* (Summer 1990): 55–79.

36. Bailin, *Sickroom in Victorian Fiction*, 6.

37. Ibid., 7.

38. My theory of health and the role of maintenance aligns with a recently published edited collection by Caroline Levine and Mario Ortiz-Robles, *Narrative Middles: Navigating the Nineteenth-Century Novel* (Columbus: Ohio State University Press, 2011), which focuses attention on the cultural, political, social, and narrative function of middles in British novels.

39. George Eliot, *Middlemarch* (New York: W. W. Norton, 2000).

40. For a discussion of Eliot's medical realism, see Lawrence Rothfield's *Vital Signs: Medical Realism in Nineteenth-Century Fiction* (Princeton: Princeton University Press, 1994). For a corrective of Rothfield's discussion of the history of the medical profession, see Caldwell, *Literature and Medicine*, 6–8.

41. Sir John Sinclair summarizes the "Rules for the Preservation of Life" as "1. Breathe pure air; 2. Use a moderate portion of liquid food; 3. Consume no more solid food than the stomach can easily subdue; 4. Preserve the organs of digestion in good order; 5. Take regular exercise without incurring fatigue; 6. Sleep as many hours only as may be necessary to restore the strength of the body and mind; 7. Control the passions, and bear with fortitude the disappointments of life" (*Code of Health* [1818], 350).

42. Rita Charon, *Narrative Medicine: Honoring the Stories of Illness* (Oxford: Oxford University Press, 2006).

CHAPTER 1: JANE AUSTEN'S PLOTS OF PREVENTION

1. Thomas Beddoes, *Hygeia: or, Essays Moral and Medical, on the Causes Affecting the Personal State of Our Middling and Affluent Classes*, ed. Robert Mitchell (Bristol, UK: Thoemmes Continuum, 2004).

2. See Dorothy Porter and Roy Porter, *Patient's Progress: Doctors and Doctoring in Eighteenth-Century England* (Cambridge, UK: Polity Press, 1989); and Roy Porter and Dorothy Porter, "The Rise of the English Drug Industry: The Role of Thomas Corbyn," *Medical History* 33 (1989): 280.

3. Ginnie Smith, "Prescribing the Rules of Health: Self-Help and Advice in the Late Eighteenth Century," in *Patients and Practitioners: Lay Perceptions of Medicine in Pre-industrial Society*, ed. Roy Porter (Cambridge: Cambridge University Press, 1985), 249.

4. William Buchan's *Domestic Medicine; or, A Treatise on the Prevention and Cure of Diseases by Regimen and Simple Medicines*, 17th ed. (Halifax: Abraham Hodge, 1801) had more popular appeal than did Beddoes's *Hygeia*. As C. J. Lawrence explains, from the time of its first publication in 1769, "[n]ew editions, reprints and pirated versions appeared every few years in Britain until 1846." Lawrence, "William Buchan: Medicine Laid Open," *Medical History* 19, no. 1 (1975): 20. *Domestic Medicine*, along with Beddoes's *Hygeia* (1802–3), was part of the influx of medical manuals written for popular audiences during this period. Though Buchan and Beddoes had different attitudes toward therapeutics as it

relates to home health care, both physicians invoked prophylactic medicine as central to the medical education of the general public.

5. Wiltshire, *Jane Austen,* 9.

6. Beddoes, "Misc." in *Hygeia,* 3. In an earlier section dealing with scrofula (which he spelled "scrophula"), Beddoes argues that parents should "teac[h] children accurately to distinguish the parts of the body. Such information will lead them to observe many important changes, which as they take place slowly, are apt to proceed unobserved. It would also render them alive to sensations, that would otherwise escape attention" ("Essay VI" in *Hygeia,* 46).

7. Nina Auerbach calls Fanny a "walking ought," arguing, "Though the word 'ought' resounds in the novel, it is used anarchically, not authoritatively, for there is no objective code to endow it with validity." Auerbach, "Feeling as One Ought about Fanny Price," in *Jane Austen's* Mansfield Park, ed. Harold Bloom, Modern Critical Interpretations (New York: Chelsea House, 1987), 116. I would argue that the "ought" and Fanny get their authority from prevention.

8. The desire to locate an origin of disease in the improperly managed family hearkens back to the stories of Adam and Eve. Many medical guides refer to the Fall as the beginning of medical suffering. Wesley uses this rhetoric in his manual to explain why everyone should have equal access to medical knowledge. Before the Fall, "[man] knew no sin, so he knows no pain, no sickness, weakness, or bodily disorder." John Wesley, *Primitive Physick; or, An Easy and Natural Method of Curing Most Diseases,* 10th ed. (Bristol, UK: Printed by William Pine, 1767), iii. Wesley demonstrates how we can use medicine to live with the consequences of this rebellion.

9. See, e.g., George Cheyne, *An Essay of Health and Long Life: Aging and Old Age* (New York: Arno Press, 1979), esp. xiv.

10. Jane Austen, *Sense and Sensibility* (New York: Penguin Classics, 1995).

11. Buchan, *Domestic Medicine,* 69.

12. One could argue that Marianne's initial fall is the first preventable injury, but I do not see the fall as a conscious act in the same way that her later practices of walking in wet grass and sitting around in wet stockings are. In *Jane Austen and the Body* (46–47), John Wiltshire refers to Buchan's *Domestic Medicine* to diagnose Marianne's fever and thus to demonstrate Austen's realism—Austen's description of remitting fever follows what Buchan writes about.

13. Although the Eliza story is probably the most tragic of Austen's embedded narratives of a fallen woman, Mrs. Smith's story in *Persuasion* comes close to replicating the type of "wretch story" that prevention manuals foresee, with its similarly tragic moral and medical consequences.

14. Claudia Johnson demonstrates the extent to which Austen's novels critique the trope of the dying sentimental heroine. Johnson suggests that Colonel Brandon's "story about poor Eliza reads like an imbedded radical novel of the 1790s, arraigning the callousness of tyrannical patriarchs whose principal object in life is to repair the waning fortunes of dissipated estates." Johnson, "'Sweet

Face as White as Death': Jane Austen and the Politics of Female Sensibility," *Novel* (Winter 1989): 167. I would add that the initial Eliza tale, with its negligent parenting and consumptive ending, resonates with the discourse of prevention as well as the discourse of sentimentality that Johnson sees structuring the parallel between Marianne and Eliza. Sentimentality and certainly melodrama are components of the prevention narrative.

15. Beddoes, "Essay I" in *Hygeia,* 84.

16. Jane Austen, *Mansfield Park* (New York: Penguin Classics, 1996).

17. Lionel Trilling, "Mansfield Park," in *Jane Austen: A Collection of Essays,* ed. Ian Watt (Englewood Cliffs, NJ: Prentice Hall, 1963), 128.

18. In *Jane Austen and the Body,* Wiltshire notes, "Fanny Price is the only one of Jane Austen's heroines whose body is frail, 'debilitated' or 'enfeebled' and, partly because of this, the character is notoriously an obstacle to the appreciation of *Mansfield Park.*" He goes on to argue, "One way round the obstacle of Fanny Price's unloveableness is to think of her as a study in developmental psychology, in the power of formative influences" (63). Wiltshire provides a compelling analysis of Fanny's psychosocial and sexual development—the way her body manifests her repressed and transgressive desire—but my focus on the way Fanny's debility marks her as an agent of prevention challenges the type of reading that emphasizes her development and growth.

19. Lorri G. Nandrea, "Difference and Repetition in Austen's *Persuasion,*" *Studies in the Novel* 39, no. 1 (2007): 49.

20. Nicholas Dames, "Austen Nostalgics," *Representations* 73 (2001): 121.

21. Critics interpret Fanny's physical condition in various ways. Laurie Kaplan and Richard Kaplan, M.D., note, "Fanny Price may simply be anemic." Kaplan and Kaplan, "What Is Wrong with Marianne? Medicine and Disease in Jane Austen," *Persuasions: Journal of the Jane Austen Society of North America* 12 (1990): 117. In general, critics view Fanny's invalidism as psychosomatic and representative of a variety of sexual and social anxieties. In *Jane Austen and the Body,* Wiltshire suggests that Fanny's physical status reflects her social position and is symptomatic of her repressed sexuality or thwarted desire. Tony Tanner suggests that it functions as a form of "resistance against the corrosive unfettered impulse of change." Tanner, "Jane Austen and 'the Quiet Thing'—a Study of *Mansfield Park,*" in *Critical Essays on Jane Austen,* ed. B. C. Southam (London: Routledge and Kegan Paul, 1968), 149. Gloria Sybil Gross reads her as simply manipulative. Gross, "Flights into Illness: Some Characters in Jane Austen," in *Literature and Medicine during the Eighteenth Century,* ed. Marie Mulvey Roberts and Roy Porter (London: Routledge, 1993), 188–99.

22. Buchan, *Domestic Medicine,* 48.

23. Thomas Beddoes, *A Guide for Self Preservation, and Parental Affection; or, Plain Directions for Enabling People to Keep Themselves and Their Children Free From Common Disorders* (Bristol, UK: Bulgin and Rosser, 1793), 9.

24. Wiltshire suggests, too, that the illness brings Tom and Fanny closer together. Both are away from home, yearning to come back: "Fanny brought so low by anxiety and loneliness at Portsmouth, Tom by illness and the desertion of his friends at Newmarket, The pair are also linked by the way Fanny's response to the news of Maria's adultery replicates the symptoms of his fever" (*Jane Austen and the Body*, 105).

25. Beddoes, "Essay II" in *Hygeia*, 35.

26. Beddoes, "Essay XI" in ibid., 96.

27. Lloyd W. Brown, "The Comic Conclusion in Jane Austen's Novels," *PMLA* 84, no. 6 (October 1969): 1582.

28. Tanner, *Jane Austen*, 172.

29. Ibid., 173.

CHAPTER 2: HEALTH, IDENTITY, AND NARRATIVE AUTHORITY IN *Jane Eyre*

Chapter epigraphs: Bernhard Christoph Faust, *The Catechism of Health, Selected and Translated from the German of Dr. Faust* (Edinburgh: Stirling and Kenney, 1828), 3; Charlotte Brontë, *Jane Eyre* (London: Penguin Classics, 2006).

1. Faust's *Catechism of Health*, first published in Germany as a textbook for schoolchildren in 1792, was translated into several languages throughout the eighteenth and early nineteenth centuries. The first London edition was published in 1794; according to James Frederick Rogers, "a reprinting (in abbreviated form) appeared in Brooklyn as late as 1882." Rogers, "A Patron Saint and Her Agent," *American Journal of Public Health* 42, no. 9 (1952): 1100.

2. Though *Jane Eyre* earned many favorable reviews at the time, some of Brontë's contemporaries found the heroine too proud, and, as Elizabeth Rigby famously does, deem Jane's lack of gratitude reprehensible: "[S]he thanks nobody, least of all Him." Rigby, reviews of *Vanity Fair*, by William Makepeace Thackeray, and *Jane Eyre*, by Charlotte Brontë, *Quarterly Review* 83 (1848), in *Jane Eyre: An Authoritative Text, Contexts, Criticism*, edited by Richard Dunn (New York: Norton, 2001): 452. Peter Allen Dale focuses attention on the exchange between Jane and Brocklehurst, suggesting, "Th[e] question of what one might do to avoid damnation (or achieve salvation) is very much at the center of the novel, and . . . it implies the narrative's essential structure of expectation, the end toward which the narrative is assumed to be headed." Dale, "Charlotte Brontë's 'Tale Half Told': The Disruption of Narrative Structure in *Jane Eyre*," *Modern Language Quarterly* 47 (1986): 112. My focus on Jane's answer, rather than Brocklehurst's question, shifts the emphasis from salvation (the end) and religious gratitude to more secular concerns of the body and preventive strategies they invoke, for as Roy and Dorothy Porter argue in *In Sickness and in Health*, by the eighteenth century, "[t]he way of the Cross seem[ed] to have receded to

a degree that Christians of earlier centuries would have found shocking. Good health move[d] in to take its place" (21).

3. For the medical history of the Brontës, see Marianne Thormählen, ed., *The Brontës in Context* (Cambridge: Cambridge University Press, 2012), especially Janis McLarren Caldwell's chapter on physical health.

4. Sally Shuttleworth, *Charlotte Brontë and Victorian Psychology* (Cambridge: Cambridge University Press, 1996), 27.

5. Faust, *Catechism of Health,* 11 (emphasis added).

6. Fothergill, *Maintenance of Health*, 23–24.

7. Shlomith Rimmon-Kenan notes that "an affinity between 'narrative' and 'identity' has been suggested in many disciplines," that "we lead our lives as stories, and our identity is constructed both by stories we tell ourselves and others about ourselves and by the master narratives that consciously or unconsciously serve as models for ours." Rimmon-Kenan, "The Story of 'I': Illness and Narrative Identity," *Narrative* 10, no. 1 (January 2002): 11.

8. Joseph Allen Boone, *Tradition Counter Tradition: Love and the Form of Fiction* (Madison: University of Wisconsin Press, 1982), xxii.

9. Ibid., esp. 97.

10. Several critics, as Robyn Warhol notes, "read Brontë's texts as participating in feminist resistance to monologism and closure." Warhol, "Double Gender, Double Genre in *Jane Eyre* and *Villette,*" *SEL* 36, no. 4 (1996): 859. Shuttleworth argues, "The history [Jane] offers is that of a series of moments of conflict, a series, moreover, which does not display the characteristics of progression, but rather the endless reiteration of the same" (*Charlotte Brontë,* 159).

11. Medical writers note repeatedly that where we live (the climate, especially) is as important as the activities we engage in (or refrain from), the foods we eat, and the clothes we wear. "Among the most powerful agents in affecting [the] health of nations and individuals is," J. H. Walsh argues, "the state of the atmosphere we breathe." Walsh, *A Manual of Domestic Medicine and Surgery, with a Glossary of the Terms Used Therein* (London: Routledge, 1858), 4.

12. Bailin, *Sickroom in Victorian Fiction,* 48.

13. Ibid., 49.

14. Jane's role as reader and storyteller and the relationship between narrative and identity, text and body have been examined throughout several decades of criticism. See, especially, Sandra M. Gilbert and Susan Gubar, "A Dialogue of Self and Soul: Plain Jane's Progress," in *The Madwoman in the Attic: The Woman Writer and the Nineteenth-Century Literary Imagination,* 2nd ed., Yale Nota Bene (New Haven, CT: Yale University Press, 2000); and Mark Hennelly, "Jane Eyre's Reading Lessons," *ELH* 52, no. 4 (Winter 1984): 693–717. Numerous critics have focused on Brontë's interest in phrenology and physiognomy as forms of reading and their significance in her novels. See Helen Cooper's introduction to *Villette,* by Charlotte Brontë (London: Penguin Classics, 2004), xxxviii–xl; and Mary A.

Armstrong's "Reading A Head: Jane Eyre, Phrenology, and the Homoerotics of Legibility," *Victorian Literature and Culture* 33, no. 1 (2005): 107–32.

15. The terms *sick, ill,* and *disease* are depicted as synonymous. Samuel Johnson's primary definition for *sick* is "Afflicted with disease," for *illness*, "1. Badness or inconvenience of any kind, natural or moral. . . . 2. [S]ickness; malady; disorder of health" (1046). Johnson, *A Dictionary of the English Language: A Digital Edition of the 1755 Classic by Samuel Johnson,* edited by Brandi Besalke (last modified February 16, 2013). In 1988, medical anthropologist Arthur Kleinman asserted a distinction between illness and disease that is now widely accepted: "Illness refers to how the sick person and members of the family or wider social network perceive, live with, and respond to symptoms of disability," whereas "[d]isease . . . is what the practitioner creates in the recasting of illness in terms of theories of disorder." Kleinman, *Illness Narratives: Suffering, Healing, and the Human Condition* (New York: Basic Books, 1988), 3, 5.

16. Johnson, *Dictionary* (London, 1755).

17. In *City of Health,* Martin Wallen makes a similar observation, suggesting that medical writers such as Beddoes sought to affirm the opposition between health and illness by undermining theories (specifically, those of John Brown) that depict health and disease as different degrees of the same condition (esp. see chapter 3).

18. Arthur L. Caplan, "The Concepts of Health, Illness, and Disease," in *Companion Encyclopedia of the History of Medicine,* ed. W. F Bynum and Roy Porter (New York: Routledge, Taylor and Francis, 1993), 2:233–48.

19. The four humors (black bile, yellow bile, phlegm, and blood) were linked with the four elements or physical conditions: heat, cold, dryness, and moistness. Each humor was also aligned with a major organ: phlegm/brain, blood/heart, yellow bile/liver, and black bile/spleen. By the nineteenth century, medical science was more concerned with the organs than with fluids (humors), but the notion of balance and moderation established by the Greeks always resonated (and still does) with advice about maintaining health.

20. Gilbert, *Citizen's Body,* 8.

21. James, *Medicinal Dictionary,* lxvi.

22. Fothergill, *Maintenance of Health,* 3.

23. Strange, *Seven Sources of Health,* xvii.

24. Walsh, *Manual of Domestic Medicine.*

25. Fothergill, *Maintenance of Health,* 2.

26. Social critics, physicians, political writers, and novelists often equate health with social acceptability ("normalcy") and endorse a particular political view. See George C. Grinnell, "Thomas Beddoes and the Physiology of Romantic Medicine," *Studies in Romanticism* 45, no. 2 (Summer 2006): 223–50, in which he argues that health, like Judith Butler's conception of gender, is discursively produced: "Normative notions of health produce a healthy bourgeois subject primarily by forcefully producing others as infirm" (225). See also Alborn, "Normal Bodies, Normal Prices"; and Shuttleworth, *Charlotte Brontë,* esp. 151.

27. Shuttleworth, *Charlotte Brontë*, 149. In chapter 5, Shuttleworth focuses on medical beliefs about menstruation and the exertion of energy.

28. Ibid., 152.

29. Ibid., 153.

30. Ibid., 158.

31. Jane fits the profile of a "nervous temperament," which Strange describes (in men) as highly intelligent, imaginative, passionate, "slender and delicate," and "pale" (*Seven Sources of Health*, 24).

32. Bruce Haley notes that in the eighteenth century, diseases such as melancholy and mania were "somatic," because the "'nervous system' was strictly speaking part of the body. In the nineteenth century the term came to be also applied to a person's mental state, so a 'disease of the nervous system' could be regarded as psychic or somatic" (*Healthy Body*, 25).

33. For the complex meaning of "nerves" and "nervous breakdown" during the Victorian period, see Janet Oppenheim's *Shattered Nerves: Doctors, Patients, and Depression in Victorian England* (Oxford: Oxford University Press, 1991). As she notes, "Although, in theory, [nervous exhaustion] was not a form of mental illness, but a disorder of the nervous system, most British medical men during the nineteenth century acknowledge the difficulty in separating the two kinds of afflictions" (ibid., 6). By the end of the century, "the continuing failure to identify the physical basis for numerous neurotic illnesses encouraged a facile equation of nervous with 'emotional' or 'psychological'" (ibid., 9). Brontë's novel, though it demonstrates an acute awareness of the interdependence of the physical and the mental, allows for occasions when one need not impinge on the other in any significant way, when the body can remain healthy despite what is going on in the mind.

34. Alan Bewell, "*Jane Eyre* and Victorian Medical Geography," *ELH* 63, no. 3 (1996): 774.

35. Jane makes a similar move when discussing the "scanty supply of food" (*Jane Eyre*, 71). She begins with the general experience, and then offers her own as a testimony of gross mismanagement at Lowood.

36. Critics have noted the significance of locations to the plotting of *Jane Eyre*. Summarizing Peter Garrett's interpretation, Boone notes, "The novel's dialectical movement between geographic settings associated with extremes of passionate rebellion and spiritual repression (Gateshead and Lowood, Thornfield and Moor House) forms a virtual graph of Jane's psychological progression toward a synthesis of these strands of personality in the adult freedom of self and love that her final destination, Ferndean and marriage to her 'beloved master,' is meant to represent" (*Tradition Counter Tradition*, 97).

37. Jane is not the only example of this—Mary Ann Wilson stands out, though all too briefly, as a "comrade" in health (Brontë, *Jane Eyre*, 92). I want to thank David Namie for reminding me about Mary Ann.

38. Numerous studies deal primarily with the thematic and formal questions surrounding sanity in *Jane Eyre* and in British literature more generally. See, for example, Gilbert and Gubar's seminal *Madwoman in the Attic* and Shuttleworth's *Charlotte Bronte*, as well as Elizabeth J. Donaldson's recent "Revisiting the Corpus of the Madwoman: Further Notes toward a Feminist Disability Studies Theory of Mental Illness," in *Feminist Disability Studies*, ed. Kim Q. Hall, 91–111 (Bloomington: Indiana University Press, 2011). Elaine Showalter's *Female Malady: Women, Madness, and English Culture, 1830–1980* (London: Virago Press, 1985) offers a historical perspective, examining various texts, including women's diaries and novels written by women, to help uncover the vexing connection between women and insanity. See also Oppenheim's *Shattered Nerves* and Wood's *Passion and Pathology*.

39. Critics have noted the significance of fire imagery, particularly the way it connects Bertha and Jane. See, for example, Cynthia Carlton-Ford's "Intimacy without Immolation: Fire in Jane Eyre," *Women's Studies* 15, no. 4 (1988): 375–86.

40. As Boone points out, "In *Jane Eyre* both perspectival and developmental facets of the novel's form are carefully governed by a univocal goal: Jane's achievement of a balanced, 'full' identity that attains thematic and narrative synthesis in marriage to her 'likeness,' Rochester" (*Tradition Counter Tradition*, 97). Boone notes that critics have been uncomfortable with the fact that Rochester must be maimed in order to achieve this closure.

41. Rigby, reviews of *Vanity Fair* and *Jane Eyre* in Dunn, ed., *Jane Eyre: An Authoritative Text*, 452.

42. Stevie Davies, introduction to *Jane Eyre*, by Charlotte Brontë (London: Penguin Classics, 2006), xxiv.

CHAPTER 3: QUARANTINE, SOCIAL THEORY, AND *Little Dorrit*

1. Thomas Southwood Smith took Dickens on a walking tour of a slum, which became the inspiration for Jacob's Island in *Oliver Twist*. See Nancy Aycock Metz, "Discovering a World of Suffering: Fiction and the Rhetoric of Sanitary Reform, 1840–1860," *Nineteenth-Century Contexts* 15, no. 1 (1991): 65–81.

2. Charles Dickens, *Martin Chuzzlewit*, ed. Patricia Ingham (New York: Penguin Classics, 1999), 784.

3. Janis McLarren Caldwell, "Illness, Disease, and Social Hygiene," in *Charles Dickens in Context*, ed. Sally Ledger and Holly Furneaux (Cambridge: Cambridge University Press, 2011), 344.

4. Charles Dickens, *Little Dorrit*, ed. Stephen Wall and Helen Small (New York: Penguin Classics, 2003).

5. George Yeats, "'Dirty Air': *Little Dorrit*'s Atmosphere," *Nineteenth-Century Literature* 66, no. 3 (2011): 328–54.

6. *General Board of Health, Report on Quarantine* (London: Clowes, 1849). While the *Report on Quarantine* was written by the "General Board of Health"

and signed by Carlisle, Ashley, Edwin Chadwick, and T. Southwood Smith, Margaret Pelling notes that "contemporary admirers were inclined to make Smith responsible for the General Board of Health's cholera and quarantine reports." Pelling, *Cholera, Fever, and English Medicine, 1825–1865* (Oxford: Oxford University Press, 1978), 10n3).

7. Quarantine was first used in Venice in 1348 to prevent the spread of bubonic plague. The first Quarantine Act in England was passed in 1710; acts were revised throughout the nineteenth century, and eventually quarantine was abolished in 1896. See medical historian Krista Maglen's "'The First Line of Defense': British Quarantine and the Port Sanitary Authorities in the Nineteenth Century," *Social History of Medicine* 15, no. 2 (2002), 426, and "'In This Miserable Spot Called Quarantine': The Healthy and the Unhealthy in Nineteenth-Century Australian and Pacific Quarantine Stations," *Science in Context* 19, no. 3 (September 2006): 317–36 for discussions of quarantinable diseases, which included plague and yellow fever. Cholera was temporarily added to the list of diseases in 1831. Beginning in 1872, "[n]on-quarantinable infectious diseases" (specifically, "smallpox, typhoid, scarlet fever, and measles") were subject to an "alternat[iv]e system of coastal disease prevention." Maglen, "First Line of Defense," 414.

8. Hepworth Dixon, review of *Little Dorrit*, by Charles Dickens, *Athenaeum* (December 1, 1855): 1394.

9. As Maglen explains, "Quarantine was feared because it could mean that healthy passengers were confined on board a vessel with patients infected with contagious disease" ("First Line," 415–16). Charles Maclean, an early opponent of quarantine, argued in the first half of the nineteenth century that quarantine caused "19/20 of all epidemics by enforcing confinement in pestilential air; producing concealment of the disease, desertion of the sick, and deadly terror" (quoted in ibid., 417). Dr. Thomas Southwood Smith lodged a similar complaint. Following sanitationist logic, he argued, "Instead of guarding against and preventing disease, [quarantine] fosters and concentrates it . . . produc[ing] the very calamity which it endeavours to prevent" (*Report on Quarantine*, 61).

10. Dixon, review of *Little Dorrit*, 1394.

11. For a discussion of quarantine and prison metaphors, see John R. Reed, "Confinement and Character in Dickens' Novels," *Dickens Studies Annual* 1 (1970): 41–54.

12. Charles Dickens, *Pictures from Italy*. London: Bradbury and Evans, 1846

13. Trey Philpotts's note on Dickens's experience in quarantine is misleading. In his *Companion to* Little Dorrit, Philpotts explains that in *Pictures from Italy*, "Dickens describes the heat and discomfort of his own one-day experience" (45). The bulk of Dickens's description, however, makes quarantine seem rather enjoyable. This makes more sense when read in terms of *Little Dorrit*.

14. In *Charles Dickens's Networks* (Oxford: Oxford University Press, 2012), Jonathan Grossman suggests, "While, as Dickens shows, there are countless

ways that people are connected—economic, familial, romantic—the umbrella figuration (besides imprisonment) for perceiving people linked together internationally in *Little Dorrit* is as 'fellow travellers'" (194).

15. See Erwin H. Ackernecht's "Anticontagionism between 1821–1867," reprinted in *Journal of International Epidemiology* 38, no. 1 (2009): 7–21. For a complete history of maritime quarantine, see Maglen, "First Line of Defense" and Mark Harrison's *Contagion: How Commerce Has Spread* (New Haven: Yale University Press, 2013).

16. Though certainly not opposed to cleanliness, contagionists argued that minute particles ("contagia") caused disease and that contact between people or affected articles spread it. George Rosen, "Disease, Debility, and Death," in *The Victorian City*, ed. H. J. Dyos (London: Routledge and Kegan Paul, 1973), 635. The fundamental principle of quarantine was the assumption that contact between people spread disease and that only keeping sick bodies apart from healthy ones through quarantine would prevent illness and thus save lives. Southwood Smith and other anticontagionist reformers, such as Edwin Chadwick, recognized that certain diseases were contagious but argued that epidemic diseases were the result of filthy, overcrowded, poorly ventilated environments, not individual contact (or at least not contact alone). As Smith explains in his earlier treatment of the topic, "Contagion and Sanitary Laws" (January 1825), smallpox, measles, and venereal disease are known to be contagious because they "prevai[l] by the communication from person to person of that specific animal poison from which the malady derives its existence." Southwood Smith, "Contagion and Sanitary Laws," in *Public Health in the Victorian Age: Debates on the Issue from 19th Century Critical Journals*, ed. Ruth G. Hodgkinson (Farnborough, UK: Gregg, 1973), 135. "An Epidemic disease," in contrast, such as plague, yellow fever, and typhus, "prevails generally over the whole, or over a large portion of the community" (ibid., 134) and "prevails through the influence of the atmosphere" (ibid., 135). The difference between contagion and miasma has to do with how one imagines the scale and manageability of people and places. Quoting Doctor William Fergusson at length in the *Second Report on Quarantine* and later in his *Epidemics Considered* lectures, Southwood Smith emphasizes that "Places, not persons, constitute the rule of [epidemic disease's] existence. Places, not persons, comprehend the whole history, the etiology of the disease. Places, not persons!" (*Second Report*, 10). Fergusson was speaking in particular of yellow fever in Africa, but by invoking this maxim ("places, not persons"), Smith attempts to allay anxieties about bodies and individuals and to reinforce the miasmatist view that environment and atmosphere are to blame for disease transmission.

17. In Southwood Smith's discussion of the way that contagion and anticontagion debates emerged throughout the nineteenth century, Christopher Hamlin notes that the either-or thinking was a necessary tool for "dismantling an opponent's naïve oversimplification rather than for presenting one's own nuanced

view." Hamlin, *Public Health and Social Justice in the Age of Chadwick: Britain, 1800–1854* (Cambridge: Cambridge University Press, 1998), 24.

18. *The Lancet* (1838/39) presented a similar anecdote ten years earlier. See J. C. McDonald, "The History of Quarantine in Britain during the Nineteenth Century," *Bulletin of History of Medicine* 25, no. 1 (January–February 1951): 31.

19. In the *Second Report on Quarantine* (1852, Smith reaffirms his position but qualifies his claims about contagion. He explains that the differences between contagion and miasma do not matter—the important point is that quarantine cannot prevent either.

20. Charles Dickens, *The Speeches of Charles Dickens*, ed. K. J. Fielding (Oxford, UK: Clarendon, 1960), 128.

21. Public health debates, particularly when they involved questions about contagion—what it meant and how it worked—were, as historians and contemporary critics of Southwood Smith have pointed out, varied and complex. Margaret Pelling explains that anticontagionists often based their theories on older versions of contagion and ignored more-nuanced ideas about contact. Pelling, "Contagion/Germ Theory/Specificity," in *Companion Encyclopedia of the History of Medicine*, ed. W. F. Bynum and Roy Porter, 2 vols. (New York: Routledge, 1993), 323. Even Smith would have to admit that, "[i]n the whole range of politics, nay, even in that of theology itself, there is no subject on which such vague notions have prevailed; none respecting which men's minds have been so completely and so generally mystified, as contagion" ("Contagion and Sanitary Laws," 135). He would spend over twenty years explaining this mystery and offering an anticontagionist argument about epidemic disease transmission to promote sanitary reform.

22. Smith, "Contagion and Sanitary Laws," 147.

23. Steven Johnson, *The Ghost Map: The Story of London's Most Terrifying Epidemic—and How It Changed Science, Cities, and the Modern World* (New York: Riverhead Books, 2006), 71–72.

24. Ibid., 173.

25. Pelling points out that germ theory only "temporarily simplified" the debates ("Contagion/Germ Theory/Specificity," 309).

26. Despite the long-standing distinction between contagionists and anti- or noncontagionists, medical professionals could not convincingly articulate a stable definition of either mode. As Hamlin points out, "The two terms [*contagion* and *miasma*] were variously and vaguely defined and used. . . . Sometimes they were used synonymously and sometimes they were answers to different questions" (*Public Health*, 60–61).

27. Margaret Pelling, "The Meaning of Contagion: Reproduction, Medicine, and Metaphor," in *Contagion: Historical and Cultural Studies*, ed. Alison Bashford and Claire Hooker (London: Routledge, 2001), 26.

28. George Rosen, *A History of Public Health* (New York: MD Publications, 1958), 288.

29. Arthur Kessel, *Air, the Environment and Public Health* (Cambridge: Cambridge University Press, 2006), 36.

30. Rosen, "Disease, Debility, and Death," 636.

31. The "English System" of quarantine was instituted in 1872. The significant difference was that nobody stayed on the ship and that the healthy were separated from the sick and allowed to leave, as long as they provided information about where they were going and could be monitored. This applied to nonquarantinable diseases (i.e., diseases that were endemic, such as smallpox and measles). See Maglen, "First Line of Defense," 424–25.

32. For discussions of the way Dickens's works move between theories of contagion and miasma, see A. Susan Williams, *The Rich Man and the Diseased Poor in Early Victorian London* (London: Macmillan, 1987), 65; and Tina Young Choi, "Narrating the Unexceptional: The Art of Medical Inquiry in Victorian England and the Present," *Literature and Medicine* 22, no. 1 (2003): 65–83.

33. Charles Dickens, *Bleak House*, ed. Nicola Bradbury (New York: Penguin Classics, 2003).

34. Mary Burgan uses *Bleak House* as a "guide" for her discussion of the differences between Victorianist and Americanist views on disease, noting, "There is nothing like *Bleak House* in American literature." Burgan, "Contagion and Culture: A View from Victorian Studies," *American Literary History* 14, no. 4 (2002): 837.

35. There are two theories about the disease that afflicts Esther: most critics assume that she contracted smallpox from Jo, while some prefer to diagnose her as suffering from erysipelas. My own reading follows from John Jordan's in *Supposing Bleak House* (Charlottesville: University of Virginia Press, 2011), which maintains the ambiguity of Esther's illness. See F. S. Schwarzbach, "The Fever of Bleak House," *English Language Notes* 20, no. 3/4 (March 1983): 21–27; and Michael S. Gurney, "Disease as Device: The Role of Smallpox in *Bleak House*," *Literature and Medicine* 9 (1990): 79–92.

36. In "*Bleak House:* The Social Pathology of Urban Life," *Literature and Medicine* 9 (1990): 93–104, F. S. Schwarzbach focuses on the meaning of fog and mud, arguing that to assume "that [they] are symbols of social malaise is to miss the point entirely: Dickens is pointing to a literal economy of filth and disease that functions . . . as fact to poison the very air the readers breathe" (95).

37. Tina Young Choi is one of the few critics who note that *Bleak House* is invested in contagionist rather than anticontagionist (miasmatist) rhetoric. Choi argues that contagionists focused on the mundane, the ordinary, and the individual, whereas the anticontagionists emphasized the extraordinary, catastrophic, and general. As Choi demonstrates, "The social logic Dickens reveals through his plot is contagionist, such that the ordinary and unremarkable actions and events are often the most consequential, and the expert knowledge of professionals is no more privileged than the observations of the layperson" ("Narrating

the Unexceptional," 76). In *Little Dorrit,* we see the range of rhetorical choices used on both sides. For discussions of contagion, see also Allan Christensen's *Nineteenth-Century Narratives of Contagion: "Our Feverish Contact"* (London: Routledge, 2005). For a discussion of disease transmission, see Nadja Durbach's *Bodily Matters: The Anti-Vaccination Movement in England, 1853–1907* (Durham, NC: Duke University Press, 2005).

38. Thomas Carlyle, *Past and Present* (New York: New York University Press, 1977), 39.

39. Ibid., 151.

40. Tina Young Choi, "Writing the Victorian City: Discourses of Risk, Connection, and Inevitability," *Victorian Studies* 43, no. 4 (2001): 571.

41. Laura Fasick argues, "In Dickens' novels . . . the trope of disease becomes a way of moving from an emphasis on social responsibility to an emphasis on personal goodness," which she describes as a shift from "body politic to body private." Fasick, "Dickens and the Diseased Body in *Bleak House,*" *Dickens Studies Annual: Essays on Victorian Fiction* 24 (1996): 137.

42. See Choi's "Writing the Victorian City" for a discussion of "risk" and the rise of "systematized statistical analysis of disease, mortality, and life expectancy for all regions of the British Isles" (572). Focusing on the discourse of sanitary reform, Choi demonstrates how "the ubiquity and unavoidability of urban filth and disease-generating miasma helped construct the Victorian city as a space in which the individual must be constantly aware, not only of the presence of others, but also of the threat of their connectedness to him or herself" (ibid., 572).

43. Although the *Report on Quarantine* was written by the General Board of Health and signed by Carlisle, Ashley, Edwin Chadwick, and T. Southwood Smith, Margaret Pelling notes, "Contemporary admirers were inclined to make Smith responsible for the General Board of Health's cholera and quarantine reports." Pelling, *Cholera, Fever, and English Medicine,* 10n3.

44. Smith, *Report on Quarantine,* 61.

45. Yeats points out, "As the title makes explicit, the idea of miasmic cholera served Dickens as an analogue for the 'moral infection' of investment in Merdle" ("Dirty Air," 334).

46. The footnote in the Penguin Classics edition for the chapter title explains, "Dickens's readers would no doubt have recalled the cholera epidemics of 1849 and 1854; also the high mortality rate from smallpox" (*Little Dorrit,* 970). Cholera and smallpox were entirely different forms of "epidemic" disease. Most Victorians believed that cholera was caused and spread by the environment. In contrast, smallpox (thanks in large part to Jenner) was known to spread by direct contact. The elision of this distinction in the footnote is similar to the elision that Dickens makes here. I do not see Dickens as conflating the ideas of disease transmission but rather shifting between the two. The effect of this slippage is to alternate

between persons and places, between individual/private and social/public responsibility at key moments in the narrative. At times the two overlap—one contributes to or exacerbates the other—but they are generally not the same.

47. Contagionists also believed that contact with things, particularly fabrics, could transmit disease. For a discussion of infectious disease and material culture, see O'Connor's *Raw Material,* 33–34. I am focusing on person-to-person contact because that is what Dickens's works, which are less interested in infected objects, draw on.

48. The article *the* in front of *contagion* suggests that Dickens is referring to the actual poison and not the theory of transmission. It is what we would now refer to as the germ or bacteria.

49. Yeats, "Dirty Air," 338.

50. Almost ten years before writing *Little Dorrit,* Dickens invoked an opposing metaphor, one based on miasma rather than contagion, in *Dombey and Son* (1846–48)(London: Penguin Books, 1985), for a similar effect. The narrator explains, "Those who study the physical sciences, and bring them to bear upon the health of Man, tell us that if the noxious particles that rise from vitiated air were palpable to the sight, we should see them lowering in a dense black cloud above such haunts, and rolling slowly on to corrupt the better portions of a town. But if the moral pestilence that rises with them and in the eternal laws of outraged Nature, is inseparable from them, could be made discernible too, how terrible the revelation!" (*Dombey and Son,* 540). In this metaphor of disease transmission, Dickens adheres to a sanitary model, highlighting air, rather than a quarantine model, which would highlight touch.

51. Chapter 1 of *Little Dorrit,* which is set in a Marseilles prison, offers a similar narrative of transmission in that Rigaud tells his story to John Baptist. This narrative, however, transmits in only one direction—Rigaud tells his story to Baptist—and therefore does not constitute the kind of connectedness and sociability we see between Arthur and Mr. Meagles.

52. Sir John Sinclair, *Code of Health and Longevity,* 4th ed. (London: McMillan, 1818), 348–49.

53. The author of an article criticizing Smith's *Report on Quarantine* and supporting quarantine nonetheless reinforces the potential danger of physical contact: "Whatever [quarantine's] defects, barbarities, and abuses, it avowedly prevents the one medium of communication (disputed, if you will) namely, touch." "Quarantine," *Fraser's Magazine* 47 (1853): 82.

54. Hilary M. Schor explains, "The narrative's own metaphor for its activity, one based on roads and prisons, comes from [Miss Wade]." Schor, *Dickens and the Daughter of the House* (Cambridge: Cambridge University Press, 1999), 129.

55. Amanda Anderson, *The Powers of Distance: Cosmopolitanism and the Cultivation of Detachment* (Princeton: Princeton University Press, 2001), 79.

56. Ibid.

57. For an extended discussion of Miss Wade and contagion as a commentary on female sexuality, see Annamarie Jagose, "Remembering Miss Wade: *Little Dorrit* and the Historicizing of Female Perversity," *GLQ* 4, no. 3 (1998): 423–51.

58. Jonathan Arac suggests, "The plague that literally terrified Marseilles metaphorically fills London's moral atmosphere." Arac, *Commissioned Spirits: The Shaping of Social Motion in Dickens, Carlyle, Melville, and Hawthorne* (New Brunswick, NJ: Rutgers University Press, 1979), 39.

59. For references to Arthur's suspicion, see Janice Carlyle, *The Sense of an Audience: Dickens, Thackeray, and George Eliot at Mid-Century* (Athens: University of Georgia Press, 1982), esp. 109–11; and Garrett Stewart, "Dickens and the Narratography of Closure," *Critical Inquiry* 34, no. 3 (Spring 2008): 518.

60. Schor explains, "What [Mrs. Clennam] wanted was Arthur's affection; if she cannot win it from his 'other mother,' she will settle for taking the other inheritance. But the story she tells leaves little doubt that if she had more love, she would need less money—and fewer documents" (*Dickens and the Daughter*, 136).

61. See Reginia Gagnier's compelling discussion of the "physiology of hope" and of *Little Dorrit* as "a novel of hope" in "Freedom, Determinism, and Hope in *Little Dorrit:* A Literary Anthropology," *Partial Answers: Journal of Literature and the History of Ideas* 9, no. 2 (2011): 331–46.

62. Reed explains that Arthur's "incarceration is a quarantine" but then focuses primarily on how his illness allows him to recognize Little Dorrit's worth: "His incarceration facilitates the intimacy with Little Dorrit that will free his spirit" ("Confinement and Character," 47).

CHAPTER 4: THE OMNISCIENCE OF INVALIDISM: THE CASE OF HARRIET MARTINEAU

1. "Invalid's Grievance," *All the Year Round* (September 10, 1887): 443.

2. Frawley, *Invalidism and Identity*, 20.

3. Ibid., 22. Frawley's comprehensive study accounts for the invalid's rising significance, arguing that a variety of forces converged—particularly during the first half of the nineteenth century—to make the invalid a recognizable and desirable (if not totally coherent) identity category. Focusing on nonfiction written by different types of invalids, Frawley demonstrates how "Evangelicalism, the emergence of an industrial national identity and a concomitant middle-class, capitalist work ethic, self-help ideology, and the 'rise' of professionalized medicine all worked in various ways to produce a climate in which the figure of the invalid could assume prominence and narratives about invalidism could prosper" (ibid., 32).

4. Criticism about narration and illness generally focuses on "nervous" patients or characters and the issue of unreliability. See Peter Melville Logan, *Nerves and Narratives: A Cultural History of Hysteria in Nineteenth-Century*

British Prose (Berkeley: University of California Press, 1997); and Katherine Snyder's section titled "Unreliability, Intelligibility, and Invalidism: *Wuthering Heights* and *Blithedale Romance*" in *Bachelors, Manhood, and the Novel, 1850–1925* (Cambridge: Cambridge University Press, 2000).

5. Harriet Martineau, *Life in the Sick-Room,* ed. Maria H. Frawley (Toronto, ON: Broadview Press, 2003), 42.

6. "Novels Past and Present," *Saturday Review* (April 14, 1866): 439.

7. Maria Frawley suggests that Gaskell is "the Victorian novelist who perhaps made the most frequent use of the invalid in her writing." Frawley, *Invalidism and Identity*, 245.

8. Arac, *Commissioned Spirits,* 3, 2.

9. Frawley, *Invalidism and Identity*, 3.

10. C.K., "On the Privileges of Invalids," *Christian Spectator,* n.s., 1 (December 1827): 632.

11. Ibid., 634.

12. In a letter to Bulwer Lytton, Harriet Martineau praised a collection of his essays entitled *The Student: A Series of Papers* (1835) and responded to his observation—or perhaps accusation—that there are similarities between a portion of that work and Martineau's recently published *Life in the Sick-Room* (1844). Addressing her response to "Dear Sir Edward," Martineau wrote,

> I like the Student the best of your earlier works. . . . It is curious,—I had ordered the Student, just two posts before your first letter came,—a fortnight since. I read it on my voyage out to America, and was much struck with it, but never saw it again, and had forgotten all about the invalidism in it,—remembering the speculations. It is very possible that the part about sickness may have dwelt in my mind, without my consciousness, and have had something to do with my late volume: but if so, it was quite unawares. (*Harriet Martineau: Selected Letters,* ed. Valerie Sanders [Oxford, UK: Clarendon Press, 1990], 82–83)

13. Edward Bulwer Lytton, "On Ill Health, and Its Consolations," in *The Student: A Series of Papers,* vol. 1 (London: Saunders and Otley, 1840), 164.

14. See, for example, some of the seminal works in this area of narrative study: Henry James, *The Art of the Novel: Critical Prefaces* (New York: Scribner and Sons, 1937); Wayne Booth, *The Rhetoric of Fiction,* 2nd ed. (Chicago: University of Chicago Press, 1983); Gerard Genette, *Narrative Discourse: An Essay in Method,* trans. Jonathan Culler (Ithaca, NY: Cornell University Press, 1983).

15. Audrey Jaffe, *Vanishing Points: Dickens, Narrative, and the Subject of Omniscience* (Berkeley: University of California Press, 1991), 4, 6.

16. Jaffe points out that critics disagree on the precise nature of the omniscient narrator, noting, "The novel critic must now choose, it seems, between

treating omniscient narrators as a presence or a personification, or an impersonal technique" (ibid., 3). Her call for an alternative that sees this type of narrator as moving among these poles is akin to how I approach the invalid and the condition of invalidism—at least as it existed during the nineteenth century.

17. Several critics have talked about *Life in the Sick-Room*'s uniqueness. Frawley suggests, "Never again would a nineteenth century British author deem it necessary or desirable to analyze chronic illness in so extended a manner" (*Invalidism and Identity*, 234). See also Alison Winter, "Harriet Martineau and the Reform of the Invalid in Victorian England," *Historical Journal* 38, no. 3 (1995): 597–616.

18. Frawley, introduction to *Life in the Sick-Room*, 11.

19. John Mullen's "Hypochondria and Hysteria: Sensibility and the Physicians" in *Sentiment and Sociability: The Language of Feeling in the Eighteenth Century* (Oxford, UK: Clarendon Press, 1988) discusses the ways in which physicians such as Cheyne and Blackmore constructed the hypochondriac in the eighteenth century as possessing a heightened sensibility. In these cases, according to Robert James's *Medicinal Dictionary* (published 1743–45), the "hypochondriacal constitution" generally referred to "those who lead a sedentary Life, and indulge themselves too much in Study" (quoted in Mullen, "Hypochondria and Hysteria"). As Mullen suggests, this malady became part of a continuum that included insanity and madness. Martineau was working against this medical view.

20. John Forster, *The Life of Charles Dickens: The Illustrated Edition*, ed. Holly Furneaux (New York: Sterling Signature, 2011), 296.

21. Frawley explains that Martineau "construct[ed] invalidism as a condition of mental activity, as opposed to physical disability" ("Prisoner to the Couch," 185). See Diana Postlethwaite, "Mothering and Mesmerism in the Life of Harriet Martineau," *Signs: Journal of Women in Culture and Society* 14, no. 3 (1989): 583–609; and Alison Winter, *Mesmerized: Powers of Mind in Victorian Britain* (Chicago: University of Chicago Press, 1998).

22. After Martineau publicized mesmerism, not medicine, as curing her condition, her brother-in-law and doctor, Thomas Greenhow, presented details about her illness in a cheap pamphlet "open," as she said, "to all the world!" (*Life in the Sick-Room*, 21). Letters published in the *Athenaeum*, presumably by Sir Benjamin Collins Brodie, attempted to discredit Martineau's claims, suggesting that she was hysterical. He argued that her lack of expertise and her status as a patient precluded her from making an accurate diagnosis of her condition (Winter, *Mesmerized*, 226).

23. Harriet Martineau, *Deerbrook*, ed. Valerie Sanders (London: Penguin, 2004).

24. Significantly, Martineau's invalids have not always been in their transcendent position. A traumatic event or a condition that develops over time defines their condition. As a result, these invalids have a sense of what it means

to be part of the world they must now primarily observe. They are defined by their sense of life before and after they have come to inhabit their current position.

25. For discussions of illness as a resistance to narrative closure, see Bailin, *Sickroom in Victorian Fiction,* 6; and Vrettos, *Somatic Fictions.*

26. Gaby Weiner, introduction to *Deerbrook,* by Harriet Martineau (Garden City, NY: Dial Press, 1984), xiv. See Deirdre David, *Intellectual Women and Victorian Patriarchy: Harriet Martineau, Elizabeth Barrett Browning, George Eliot* (New York: Cambridge University Press, 1987); and Caroline Roberts, *The Woman and the Hour: Harriet Martineau and Victorian Ideologies* (Toronto: University of Toronto Press, 2002).

27. Valerie Sanders, *Reason over Passion: Harriet Martineau and the Victorian Novel* (Sussex, UK: Harvester Press, 1986), 60.

28. Ibid., 92–93.

29. Gillian Thomas, *Harriet Martineau,* Twayne's English Author Series (Boston: Twayne, 1985), 113.

30. As many critics have noted, Martineau made strong claims about the disadvantages of marriage for a woman like herself. See Harriet Martineau, *Autobiography,* ed. Maria Weston Chapman (Boston: James R. Osgood and Company, 1877). See also Florence Nightingale's *Cassandra: An Essay* (Old Westbury, NY: Feminist Press, 1979), which explicitly invokes invalidism as a way to remove women from the drudgery of domestic duty but also condemns the current social conditions for creating passive women.

31. Charlotte M. Yonge developed such figures in her fiction later in the century, most notably Ermine Williams in *The Clever Woman of the Family,* ed. Clare A. Simmons (1865; Peterborough, ON: Broadview Press, 2001).

32. In a chapter entitled "Some Gains and Sweets of Invalidism," Martineau writes, "Where there is a habit of mutability, there is intellectual infirmity, as is shown, with indescribable clearness, to us gazers in the mirror of events" (*Life in the Sick-Room,* 157). Maria Frawley suggests that Martineau constructed the invalid in *Life in the Sick-Room* as "in control of the 'gaze' that some theorists believe divests the clinical patient of individuality and a sense of self" (*Invalidism and Identity,* 228). Caroline Roberts explores the function of the clinical gaze in *Deerbrook,* noting that unlike Hester and Margaret, Maria is never subject to its control (*Woman and the Hour,* 74). Neither critic notes ways in which the gaze reverberates in both texts.

33. Critics have noted Martineau's connection to Romanticism in both *Deerbrook* and *Life in the Sick-Room.* See David, *Intellectual Women;* and Deborah Logan, *The Hour and the Woman: Harriet Martineau's "Somewhat Remarkable Life"* (Dekalb: Northern Illinois University Press, 2002), 26.

34. David reads this scene as autobiographical, noting that reading Milton and "overlooking people . . . are Martineau's pleasures" (*Intellectual Women,* 83).

35. Manfred Jahn discusses the role of interior monologues in the works of Gerard Genette and Dorrit Cohn, who describe the "monologist" as a "'substitute' narrator." Jahn, "Windows of Focalization: Deconstructing and Reconstructing a Narratological Concept," *Style* 30, no. 2 (1996): 247.

36. Mrs. Enderby (Philip and Mrs. Rowland's mother) suffers from unspecified attacks that physically and mentally drain her. Like Maria, Mrs. Enderby enjoys observing from her window. At one point, she asks her grandchildren to "make a snow-man in [the] field," so she can "sit here and watch" and "think [they] are saying something kind to [her]" (Martineau, *Deerbrook*, 189). I do not treat Mrs. Enderby more fully, because she functions primarily as a plot device and a means for revealing Mrs. Rowland's evil machinations. Although there are parallels between Maria and Mrs. Enderby, the narrator focalizes our reading through Maria. Moreover, the parallels between *Life in the Sick-Room* and *Deerbrook* revolve around Maria's perspective rather than Mrs. Enderby's.

37. Focusing on the tension in Martineau's writing between privacy and openness, particularly in the context of her commentary on the bank failures of the 1830s, Aeron Hunt argues that Martineau's depiction of Maria's narratorial role and the speculation that comes with it demonstrate an "underlying concern that perhaps the practice of probing . . . private matters and feelings is not entirely savory." Hunt, "Open Accounts: Harriet Martineau and the Problem of Privacy in Early-Victorian Culture," *Nineteenth-Century Literature* 62, no. 1 (2007): 27.

38. Frawley, "Prisoner to the Couch," 184. Frawley also notes that the window "marks the invalid's access to the wider world" and "signif[ies] the meditative and visionary powers of invalidism" (ibid., 183).

39. Diana Postlethwaite notes the parallels between Martineau looking out of her sickroom window with her telescope and Dorothea Brooke of *Middlemarch* "looking out her window at the sunrise to 'the largeness of the world and the manifold wakings of men to labour and endurance'" ("Mothering and Mesmerism," 603).

40. Frawley describes Martineau as an "invalid ethnographer, filling volumes with what she observes, creating samples, and analyzing her findings" ("Prisoner to the Couch," 184).

41. Valerie Kossow Pichanick describes Maria as "suffering from an anguished and humiliating unrequited passion" (*Harriet Martineau: The Woman and Her Work, 1802–1876* [Ann Arbor: University of Michigan Press, 1980], 117), whereas Valerie Sanders calls her "the first in a long sad line of drearily unfortunate governesses" (*Reason over Passion*, 60).

42. In her *Autobiography* (1877), Martineau writes,

> My strong will, combined with anxiety of conscience, makes me fit only to live alone; and my taste and liking are for living alone. The older I have grown, the more serious and irremediable have seemed to

> me the evils and disadvantages of married life, as it exists among us at this time: and I am provided with what it is the bane of single life in ordinary cases to want,—substantial, laborious and serious occupation. My business in life has been to think and learn, and to speak out with absolute freedom what I have thought and learned. (101–2)

43. Martineau criticizes a religion that, "proud of its Christian faith as the 'Worship of Sorrow,' thinks it a duty and a privilege to dwell on the morbid conditions of human life" (*Autobiography*, 432).

CHAPTER 5: NARRATIVE COMPETENCE AND THE FAMILY DOCTOR IN GASKELL'S *Wives and Daughters*

1. Cheyne, *Essay of Health and Long Life*, 5.

2. Dorothy Porter and Roy Porter discuss the role of patient narratives in Georgian medicine, noting that "a sick person would write to an eminent physician enclosing his own medical history; the physician's reply would include diagnosis, directions for a regimen and a prescription to be made up by the local apothecary or druggist, or, if simple, at home. In following this procedure, the patient was expected . . . to internalize the doctor." (*Patient's Progress*, 76). These narratives were replaced in the nineteenth century by the physical exam. Gaskell's *Wives and Daughters* demonstrates both a nostalgia for and an anticipation of story-based diagnostics and therapy.

3. See Tabitha Sparks, *The Doctor in the Victorian Novel: Family Practice* (Aldershot, UK: Ashgate, 2009).

4. Sydney Smith criticizes Martineau's choice of a doctor hero (quoted in Vineta Colby, *Yesterday's Woman: Domestic Realism in the English Novel* [Princeton: Princeton University Press, 1974], 213.

5. Elizabeth Gaskell, *Wives and Daughters* (London: Penguin, 1996).

6. Anthony Trollope's Dr. Thorne (*Doctor Thorne*, Chronicles of Barsetshire [London: Chapman and Hall, 1858]) is another notable precursor to Dr. Gibson, though his practice is fraught in numerous ways that add to the novel's humor and suspense. Not only does Thorne regularly argue in the periodical press with his medical peers, but also he is the only character privy to the secret identity of his patient's heir.

7. See Marie Fitzwilliam, "Mr Harrison's Confessions: A Study of the General Practitioner's Social and Professional Dis-Ease," *Gaskell Society Journal* 12 (1998): 28–36.

8. Hilary M. Schor, *Scheherezade in the Marketplace: Elizabeth Gaskell and the Victorian Novel* (New York: Oxford University Press, 1992), 187.

9. This kind of heroine appeared later in the century as the New Woman. Charlotte Yonge represents a failed version of the new woman in *Clever Woman of the Family*, published the same year as *Wives and Daughters*. In this story,

Rachel Curtis dabbles in medicine but ends up killing a young girl with one of her holistic remedies. She learns by the end of the novel that it is better to be married and not so clever.

10. See Rita Charon, "Narrative Medicine: A Model for Empathy, Reflection, Profession, and Trust," *JAMA* 286, no. 1 (October 17, 2001): 1897–1902.

11. Roy Porter explains that Beddoes valued his patient's stories: "It has long been my custom to request a particular narrative, in writing of all circumstances which they suppose to have any relation to their complaint." Beddoes quoted in Roy Porter, *Doctor of Society: Thomas Beddoes and the Sick Trade in Late Enlightenment England,* The Wellcome Institute Series in the History of Medicine (London: Routledge, 1992), 45. Beddoes thought that all data from doctors should be "systematically preserved for public consultation" (ibid., 46). He proposed a "more energetic medical publication" and "more systematic collection and indexing of medical facts in convenient archives" (ibid., 46). A good physician, Beddoes believed, must be a good listener (ibid., 77–78).

12. Critics have noted the important ways in which Mr. Gibson's profession reinforces the novel's interest in evolutionary science; his interest in medical science is part of a larger narrative of progress and masculine knowledge. See Schor, *Scheherezade in the Marketplace;* Deirdre D'Albertis, *Dissembling Fictions: Elizabeth Gaskell and the Victorian Social Text* (New York: St. Martin's, 1997); Leon Litvack, "Outposts of Empire: Scientific Discovery and Colonial Displacement in Gaskell's *Wives and Daughters,*" *Review of English Studies: The Leading Journal of English Literature and the English Language* 55, no. 222 (2004): 727–58. My reading isolates medicine and the profession from science.

13. For a discussion of the significance of Mr. Gibson's Scottishness and medical training, see Julia Wright, "'Growing Pains': Representing the Romantic in Gaskell's *Wives and Daughters,*" in *Nervous Reactions: Victorian Recollections of Romanticism,* ed. Joel Faflak and Julia M. Wright, 163–88 (Albany: State University of New York Press, 2004).

14. As Schor notes, "The lesson of the dead mother, and the few living mother figures in the novel, is that to be female is primarily to be an invalid, to be passive, to suffer victimization. This is what both [Cynthia and Molly] try to overcome" (*Scheherazade in the Marketplace,* 190).

15. Susan Morgan, *Daughters in Time: Imagining Gender in 19th-Century British Fiction* (Oxford: Oxford University Press, 1989), 112.

16. Ibid., 113.

17. Ibid., 112.

18. Gaskell explores the dangers of such parental ignorance in *Cousin Phillis* (1864), published in *Cornhill* just prior to *Wives and Daughters.* In this novella, the parents' inability to see that their daughter has outgrown her pinafores, that she is a woman capable of romantic love, almost kills her.

19. Elizabeth Langland, *Nobody's Angels: Middle-Class Women and Domestic Ideology in Victorian Culture* (Ithaca, NY: Cornell University Press, 1995), 137.

20. Schor, *Scheherezade in the Marketplace*, 187.

21. Written ten years before *Mary Barton*, the diary has been considered by some to be Gaskell's "first sustained effort as a writer." Deirdre D'Albertis, "The Life and Letters of E. C. Gaskell," in *The Cambridge Companion to Elizabeth Gaskell*, ed. Linda K. Hughes (Cambridge: Cambridge University Press, 2007), 21.

22. Elizabeth Cleghorn Gaskell, *My Diary: The Early Years of My Daughter Marianne* (1835–38), ed. Clement King Shorter (London: Privately printed, 1923), 6.

23. Andrew Combe, *The Principles of Physiology Applied to the Preservation of Health, and to the Improvement of Mental and Physical Education* (New York: Harper and Brothers, 1834).

24. Margaret Homans convincingly interprets Molly as "a receiver of secrets" and "selfless mediator," but her assertion that "Molly begins to shift from the language of one kind of mother to that of the other" ignores the way Molly adopts and adapts her father's language of medicine. Homans, *Bearing the Word: Language and Female Experience in Nineteenth-Century Women's Writing*, Women in Culture and Society (Chicago: University of Chicago Press, 1986), 256, 259.

25. It is worth noting that whereas Cynthia's story depends in large part on Molly's reactions to it, we get pieces of her past outside of Molly's perspective that help us develop our own expertise of Cynthia's case. In a bit of gossip, Miss Hornblower hints—though somewhat unwittingly—at a romantic triangle involving the mother and daughter. In her comments to Miss Browning about Cynthia's womanly appearance, Miss Hornblower corroborates that Cynthia was, even as a young girl, rather beautiful. Her age kept "people" from assuming that there was an inappropriate relationship, and shortly after this history, we learn of Mrs. Gibson's past involvement with Preston. Though she may be "condescending" now, Mrs. Hornblower complains, there was a time when Mrs. Kirkpatrick "would have been glad enough to marry Mr. Preston" (Gaskell, *Wives and Daughters*, 283). This exchange exposes an uncomfortable competition between mother and daughter that explains, in part, Hyacinth's desire to leave Cynthia behind or send her away. Molly learns much later, during Cynthia's confession, about Mrs. Kirkpatrick's "desperate" advances toward Mr. Preston. Oddly, this is the only time Cynthia comes to her mother's defense—when she learns from her schoolmate that people joke about "the very pretty widow . . . who made love to him," she becomes even more disgusted by her attachment to "that man" (ibid., 472). This part of the story ceases to matter, however, as Cynthia's and Molly's plots overlap through their common, though different, interest in Roger.

AFTERWORD

1. Galen, *Hygiene*, 5.

2. Gerald Prince, "Narrative Analysis and Narratology," *New Literary History* 13, no. 2 (Winter 1982): 181.

3. Charon, "Narrative Medicine," 1897.

4. Ibid. See also Kathryn Montgomery Hunter, *Doctor's Stories: The Narrative Structure of Medical Knowledge* (Princeton: Princeton University Press, 1991); Tricia Greenhalgh and Brian Hurwitz, *Narrative-Based Medicine: Dialogue and Discourse in Clinical Practice* (London: BMJ Books, 1998); and Charon, *Narrative Medicine*.

5. For an overview of this history, see Lindsay Holmgren, Abraham Fuks, Donald Boudreau, Tabitha Sparks, and Martin Kreiswirth, "Terminology and Praxis: Clarifying the Scope of Narrative in Medicine," *Literature and Medicine* 29, no. 2 (2011): 246–73.

6. In fall 2009, Columbia University began offering an MS in narrative medicine. See also www.narrativemedicine.org/links.html for links to current programs in the medical humanities.

7. Such competence, although it applies in very significant ways to the doctor-patient relationship, is also essential, as Charon points out in the *JAMA* article on "Narrative Medicine: A Model for Empathy, Reflection, and Trust," to the physician's relationship to herself, to her colleagues, and to society.

8. See Rimmon-Kenan, "The Story of 'I'"; and Arthur Frank, "The Rhetoric of Self-Change: Illness Experience as Narrative," *Sociological Quarterly* 34, no. 1 (1993): 39–52 and "Asking the Right Question about Pain: Narrative and Phronesis," *Literature and Medicine* 23, no. 2 (Fall 2004): 209–25.

Bibliography

Ackernecht, Erwin H. "Anticontagionism between 1821–1867." Reprinted in *Journal of International Epidemiology* 38, no. 1 (2009): 7–21.

Alborn, Timothy. "Normal Bodies, Normal Prices in Victorian Life Insurance." *RaVon* 49 (February 2008).

Anderson, Amanda. *The Powers of Distance: Cosmopolitanism and the Cultivation of Detachment.* Princeton: Princeton University Press, 2001.

Arac, Jonathan. *Commissioned Spirits: The Shaping of Social Motion in Dickens, Carlyle, Melville, and Hawthorne.* New Brunswick, NJ: Rutgers University Press, 1979.

Armstrong, Mary A. "Reading A Head: Jane Eyre, Phrenology, and the Homoerotics of Legibility." *Victorian Literature and Culture* 33, no. 1 (2005): 107–32.

Auerbach, Nina. "Feeling as One Ought about Fanny Price." In *Jane Austen's* Mansfield Park, edited by Harold Bloom, 103–16. Modern Critical Interpretations. New York: Chelsea House, 1987.

Austen, Jane. *Mansfield Park.* New York: Penguin Classics, 1996.

———. *Sense and Sensibility.* New York: Penguin Classics, 1995.

Bagehot, Walter. "The Waverly Novels." In *The Collected Works of Walter Bagehot,* edited by Norman St. John–Stevas. Cambridge, MA: Harvard University Press, 1965.

Bailin, Miriam. *The Sickroom in Victorian Fiction: The Art of Being Ill.* Cambridge: Cambridge University Press, 1995.

Barrett, E. B. "Little Dorrit and the Disease of Modern Life." *Nineteenth-Century Fiction* 25, no. 2 (1910): 199–215.

Beddoes, Thomas. *A Guide for Self Preservation, and Parental Affection; or, Plain Directions for Enabling People to Keep Themselves and Their Children Free from Common Disorders.* Bristol, UK: Bulgin and Rosser, 1793.

———. *Hygeia; or, Essays Moral and Medical, on the Causes Affecting the Personal State of Our Middling and Affluent Classes.* Edited by Robert Mitchell. Bristol, UK: Thoemmes Continuum, 2004.

———. *Manual of Health; or, Conducting the Invalid Safely through the Seasons.* London: Johnson, 1806.

Bewell, Alan. "*Jane Eyre* and Victorian Medical Geography." *ELH* 63 no. 3 (1996): 773–808.

Blair, Kirstie. "Pathologizing the Victorians." *Interdisciplinary Literary Studies: A Journal of Criticism and Theory* 3, no. 2 (2002): 138–43.

Boone, Joseph Allen. *Tradition Counter Tradition: Love and the Form of Fiction.* Madison: University of Wisconsin Press, 1982.

Booth, Wayne. *The Rhetoric of Fiction.* 2nd ed. Chicago: University of Chicago Press, 1983.

Brontë, Charlotte. *Jane Eyre.* London: Penguin Classics, 2006.

———. *Jane Eyre.* Edited by Richard J. Dunn. New York: Norton, 2001.

Brontë, Emily. *Wuthering Heights.* London: Penguin Classics, 2003.

Brooks, Peter. *Reading for the Plot: Design and Intention in Narrative.* Cambridge, MA: Harvard University Press, 1984.

Brown, Lloyd W. "The Comic Conclusion in Jane Austen's Novels." *PMLA* 84, no. 6 (October 1969): 1582.

Buchan, William. *Domestic Medicine; or, A Treatise on the Prevention and Cure of Diseases by Regimen and Simple Medicines.* 17th ed. Halifax: Abraham Hodge, 1801.

Burgan, Mary. "Contagion and Culture: A View from Victorian Studies." *American Literary History* 14, no. 4 (2002): 837–44.

Butler, Marilyn. *Jane Austen and the War of Ideas.* Oxford, UK: Clarendon Press, 1975.

Buzard, James. "'The Country of the Plague': Anticulture and Autoethnography in Dickens's 1850s." *Victorian Literature and Culture* 38, no. 2 (September 2010): 413–19.

Caldwell, Janis McLarren. "Illness, Disease, and Social Hygiene." In *Charles Dickens in Context,* edited by Sally Ledger and Holly Furneaux, 343–49. Cambridge: Cambridge University Press, 2011.

———. *Literature and Medicine in Nineteenth-Century Britain: From Mary Shelley to George Eliot.* Cambridge: Cambridge University Press, 2008.

———. "Physical Health." In *The Brontës in Context,* edited by Marianne Thormählen, 335–43. Cambridge: Cambridge University Press, 2012.

Caplan, Arthur L. "The Concepts of Health, Illness, and Disease." In *Companion Encyclopedia of the History of Medicine,* edited by W. F Bynum and Roy Porter, 233–48. 2 vols. New York: Routledge, Taylor and Francis, 1993.

Carlton-Ford, Cynthia. "Intimacy without Immolation: Fire in Jane Eyre." *Women's Studies* 15, no. 4 (1988): 375–86.

Carlyle, Janice. *The Sense of an Audience: Dickens, Thackeray, and George Eliot at Mid-Century.* Athens: University of Georgia Press, 1982.

Carlyle, Thomas. *Past and Present.* New York: New York University Press, 1977.

Charon, Rita. "Narrative Medicine: A Model for Empathy, Reflection, Profession, and Trust." *JAMA* 286, no. 1 (October 17, 2001): 1897–1902.

———. *Narrative Medicine: Honoring the Stories of Illness.* Oxford: Oxford University Press, 2006.

Cheyne, George. *An Essay of Health and Long Life: Aging and Old Age.* New York: Arno Press, 1979.

Choi, Tina Young. "Narrating the Unexceptional: The Art of Medical Inquiry in Victorian England and the Present." *Literature and Medicine* 22, no. 1 (2003): 65–83.

———. "Writing the Victorian City: Discourses of Risk, Connection, and Inevitability." *Victorian Studies* 43, no. 4 (2001): 561–89.

Christensen, Allan. *Nineteenth-Century Narratives of Contagion: "Our Feverish Contact."* London: Routledge, 2005.

C.K. "On the Privileges of Invalids." *Christian Spectator,* n.s., 1 (December 1827): 632–36.

Colby, Vineta. *Yesterday's Woman: Domestic Realism in the English Novel.* Princeton: Princeton University Press, 1974.

Combe, Andrew. *The Principles of Physiology Applied to the Preservation of Health, and to the Improvement of Mental and Physical Education.* New York: Harper and Brothers, 1834.

Cook, E. T., and Alexander Wedderburn, eds. Introduction to *The Works of John Ruskin,* xxiii–xlviii. London: Longmans, Green, 1908.

Cooper, Helen. Introduction to *Villette,* by Charlotte Brontë, xxxviii–xl. London: Penguin Classics, 2004.

Cooter, Roger. "The Traffic in Victorian Bodies: Medicine, Literature, and History." *Victorian Studies: An Interdisciplinary Journal of Social, Political, and Cultural Studies* 45, no. 3 (2003): 513–27.

Craik, Dinah Mulock. *John Halifax, Gentleman.* Edited by Lynn M Alexander. Peterborough, ON: Broadview, 2005.

D'Albertis, Deirdre. *Dissembling Fictions: Elizabeth Gaskell and the Victorian Social Text.* New York: St. Martin's, 1997.

———. "The Life and Letters of E. C. Gaskell." In *The Cambridge Companion to Elizabeth Gaskell,* edited by Linda K. Hughes, 10–26. Cambridge: Cambridge University Press, 2007.

Dale, Peter Allen. "Charlotte Brontë's 'Tale Half Told': The Disruption of Narrative Structure in *Jane Eyre.*" *Modern Language Quarterly* 47 (1986): 108–29.

Dames, Nicholas. "Austen Nostalgics." *Representations* 73 (2001): 117–43.

David, Deirdre. *Intellectual Women and Victorian Patriarchy: Harriet Martineau, Elizabeth Barrett Browning, George Eliot.* New York: Cambridge University Press, 1987.

Davies, Stevie. Introduction to *Jane Eyre,* by Charlotte Brontë, xi–xlii. London: Penguin Classics, 2006.

Davis, Cynthia. *Bodily and Narrative Forms: The Influence of Medicine on American Literature, 1845–1915.* Stanford: Stanford University Press, 2000.

Dickens, Charles. *Bleak House.* Edited by Nicola Bradbury. New York: Penguin Classics, 2003.

———. *Dombey and Son.* Edited by Peter Fairclough. New York: Penguin Books, 1985.

———. *Little Dorrit.* Edited by Stephen Wall and Helen Small. New York: Penguin Classics, 2003.

———. "1850 Preface." *Martin Chuzzlewit.* Edited by Patricia Ingham. New York: Penguin Classics, 1999.

———. *Master Humphrey's Clock and Other Stories.* Edited by Peter Mudford. New York: Everyman Paperback Classics, 1997.

———. *Pictures from Italy*. London: Bradbury and Evans, 1846.

———. *The Speeches of Charles Dickens.* Edited by K. J. Fielding. Oxford, UK: Clarendon, 1960.

Digby, Anne. *Making a Medical Living: Doctors and Patients in the English Market for Medicine, 1720–1911.* Cambridge Studies in Population, Economy, and Society in Past Time no. 24. Cambridge: Cambridge University Press, 1994.

Dixon, Hepworth. Review of *Little Dorrit,* by Charles Dickens. *Athenaeum* (December 1, 1855): 1393–95.

Donaldson, Elizabeth J. "Revisiting the Corpus of the Madwoman: Further Notes toward a Feminist Disability Studies Theory of Mental Illness," in *Feminist Disability Studies,* ed. Kim Q. Hall, 91–111. Bloomington: Indiana University Press, 2011.

Duckworth, Alistair. *The Improvement of the Estate: A Study of Jane Austen's Novels.* Baltimore, MD: Johns Hopkins University Press, 1994.

Durbach, Nadja. *Bodily Matters: The Anti-Vaccination Movement in England, 1853–1907.* Durham, NC: Duke University Press, 2005.

Eliot, George. *Middlemarch.* New York: W. W. Norton, 2000.

Fasick, Laura. "Dickens and the Diseased Body in *Bleak House.*" *Dickens Studies Annual: Essays on Victorian Fiction* 24 (1996): 135–51.

Faust, Bernhard Christoph. *The Catechism of Health, Selected and Translated from the German of Dr. Faust.* Edinburgh: Stirling and Kenney, 1828.

Fitzwilliam, Marie. "Mr Harrison's Confessions: A Study of the General Practitioner's Social and Professional Dis-Ease." *Gaskell Society Journal* 12 (1998): 28–36.

Forster, John. *The Life of Charles Dickens: The Illustrated Edition*. Edited by Holly Furneaux. Sterling Signature, 2011.

Fothergill, John Milner. *The Maintenance of Health: A Medical Work for Lay Readers.* London: Smith, Elder, 1874. Available from Google Books.

Frank, Arthur. "Asking the Right Question about Pain: Narrative and Phronesis." *Literature and Medicine* 23, no. 2 (Fall 2004): 209–25.

———. "The Rhetoric of Self-Change: Illness Experience as Narrative." *Sociological Quarterly* 34, no. 1(1993): 39–52.

———. Introduction to *Life in the Sick-Room,* by Harriet Martineau, 11–28. Toronto, ON: Broadview Press, 2003.

———. *Invalidism and Identity in Nineteenth-Century Britain.* Chicago: University of Chicago Press, 2004.

———. "'A Prisoner to the Couch': Harriet Martineau, Invalidism, and Self-Representation." In *The Body and Physical Difference,* edited by David T. Mitchell and Sharon L. Snyder, 174–88. Ann Arbor: University of Michigan Press, 2000.

Frawley, Maria. *Invalidism and Identity in Nineteenth-Century Britain.* Chicago: University of Chicago Press, 2004.

Gagnier, Regina. "Freedom, Determinism, and Hope in *Little Dorrit:* A Literary Anthropology." *Partial Answers: Journal of Literature and the History of Ideas* 9, no. 2 (2011): 331–46.

Galen. *Hygiene (De sanitate tuenda).* Translated by Robert Montraville Green. Introduction by Henry E. Sigerist. Springfield, IL: Charles C. Thomas, 1951.

———. *Galen: Selected Works.* Edited by P. N. Singer. Oxford World's Classics Series. Oxford: Oxford University Press, 1997.

Gaskell, Elizabeth Cleghorn. *Cranford/Cousin Phillis.* London: Penguin Classics, 1986.

———. *My Diary: The Early Years of My Daughter Marianne.* 1835–38. Edited by Clement King Shorter. London: Privately printed, 1923.

———. "Round the Sofa." *My Lady Ludlow and Other Stories,* edited by Edgar Wright. Oxford: Oxford World's Classics. 1989.

———. *Wives and Daughters.* London: Penguin, 1996.

General Board of Health, *Report on Quarantine.* London: Clowes, 1849.

———. Second Report on Quarantine. London: Clowes, 1852.

Genette, Gerard. *Narrative Discourse: An Essay in Method.* Translated by Jonathan Culler. Ithaca, NY: Cornell University Press, 1983.

Gilbert, Pamela K. *The Citizen's Body: Desire, Health, and the Social in Victorian England.* Columbus: Ohio State University Press, 2007.

———. *Disease, Desire, and the Body in Victorian Women's Popular Novels.* Cambridge: Cambridge University Press, 1997.

Gilbert, Sandra M., and Susan Gubar. *The Madwoman in the Attic: The Woman Writer and the Nineteenth-Century Literary Imagination.* 2nd ed. Yale Nota Bene. New Haven, CT: Yale University Press, 2000.

Greenhalgh, Tricia, and Brian Hurwitz. *Narrative-Based Medicine: Dialogue and Discourse in Clinical Practice.* London: BMJ Books, 1998.

Grinnell, George C. "Thomas Beddoes and the Physiology of Romantic Medicine." *Studies in Romanticism* 45, no. 2 (Summer 2006): 223–50.

Gross, Gloria Sybil. "Flights into Illness: Some Characters in Jane Austen." In *Literature and Medicine during the Eighteenth Century,* edited by Marie Mulvey Roberts and Roy Porter, 188–99. London: Routledge, 1993.

Grossman, Jonathan H. *Charles Dickens's Networks: Public Transport and the Novel.* Oxford: Oxford University Press, 2012.
Gurney, Michael S. "Disease as Device: The Role of Smallpox in *Bleak House.*" *Literature and Medicine* 9 (1990): 79–92.
Haley, Bruce. *The Healthy Body and Victorian Culture.* Cambridge, MA: Harvard University Press, 1978.
Hamlin, Christopher. *Public Health and Social Justice in the Age of Chadwick: Britain, 1800–1854.* Cambridge: Cambridge University Press, 1998.
Hennelly, Mark. "Jane Eyre's Reading Lessons." *ELH* 52, no. 4 (Winter 1984): 693–717.
Herndl, Diane Price. *Invalid Women: Figuring Feminine Illness in American Fiction and Culture, 1840–1940.* Chapel Hill: University of North Carolina Press, 1993.
Hinton, James. *Thoughts on Health and Some of Its Conditions.* London: Smith, Elder, 1871.
Holmes, Martha Stoddard. *Fictions of Affliction: Physical Disability in Victorian Culture.* Ann Arbor: University of Michigan Press, 2004.
Holmgren, Lindsay, Abraham Fuks, Donald Boudreau, Tabitha Sparks, and Martin Kreiswirth. "Terminology and Praxis: Clarifying the Scope of Narrative in Medicine." *Literature and Medicine* 29, no. 2 (2011): 246–73.
Homans, Margaret. *Bearing the Word: Language and Female Experience in Nineteenth-Century Women's Writing.* Women in Culture and Society. Chicago: University of Chicago Press, 1986.
Hunt, Aeron. "Open Accounts: Harriet Martineau and the Problem of Privacy in Early-Victorian Culture." *Nineteenth-Century Literature* 62, no. 1 (2007): 1–28.
Hunter, Kathryn Montgomery. *Doctor's Stories: The Narrative Structure of Medical Knowledge* Princeton: Princeton University Press, 1991.
"Invalid's Grievance, An." *All the Year Round* (September 10, 1887): 442–44.
Jaffe, Audrey. *Vanishing Points: Dickens, Narrative, and the Subject of Omniscience.* Berkeley: University of California Press, 1991.
Jagose, Annamarie. "Remembering Miss Wade: *Little Dorrit* and the Historicizing of Female Perversity." *GLQ* 4, no. 3 (1998): 423–51.
Jahn, Manfred. "Windows of Focalization: Deconstructing and Reconstructing a Narratological Concept." *Style* 30, no. 2 (1996): 241–66.
James, Henry. *The Art of the Novel: Critical Prefaces.* New York: Scribner and Sons, 1937.
James, Robert. *A Medicinal Dictionary.* 3 vols. London: Printed for T. Osborne, 1743–45. Eighteenth Century Collections Online. Gale. University of Southern California. Accessed 14 July 2015.
Johnson, Claudia. "'Sweet Face as White as Death': Jane Austen and the Politics of Female Sensibility." *Novel* (Winter 1989): 159–74.
Johnson, Samuel. *A Dictionary of the English Language: A Digital Edition of the 1755 Classic by Samuel Johnson.* Edited by Brandi Besalke. Last modified

February 16, 2013. Originally published London: J. and P. Knapton, 1755. http://johnsonsdictionaryonline.com.

Johnson, Steven. *The Ghost Map: The Story of London's Most Terrifying Epidemic—and How It Changed Science, Cities, and the Modern World.* New York: Riverhead Books, 2006.

Jordan, John O. *Supposing Bleak House.* Charlottesville: University of Virginia Press, 2011.

Judd, Catherine. *Bedside Seductions: Nursing and the Victorian Imagination, 1830–1880.* New York: St. Martin's Press, 1998.

Kaplan, Laurie, and Richard S. Kaplan. "What Is Wrong with Marianne? Medicine and Disease in Jane Austen." *Persuasions: Journal of the Jane Austen Society of North America* 12 (1990): 117–30.

Kennedy, Meegan. *Revising the Clinic: Vision and Representations in Victorian Medical Narratives and the Novel.* Columbus: Ohio State University Press, 2010.

Kermode, Frank. *The Sense of an Ending: Studies in the Theory of Fiction.* Oxford: Oxford University Press, 1966. Paperback edition, 2000.

Kessel, Arthur. *Air, the Environment and Public Health.* Cambridge: Cambridge University Press, 2006..

Kleinman, Arthur. *Illness Narratives: Suffering, Healing, and the Human Condition.* New York: Basic Books, 1988.

Lamb, Charles. *Elia and the Last Essays of Elia.* Edited by Jonathan Bate. Oxford: Oxford University Press, 1987.

Langland, Elizabeth. *Nobody's Angels: Middle-Class Women and Domestic Ideology in Victorian Culture.* Ithaca, NY: Cornell University Press, 1995.

Lawrence, C. J. "William Buchan: Medicine Laid Open." *Medical History* 19, no. 1 (1975): 20–35.

Levine, Caroline, and Mario Ortiz-Robles. *Narrative Middles: Navigating the Nineteenth-Century Novel.* Columbus: Ohio State University Press, 2011.

Lewes, G. H. "Training in Relation to Health." *Cornhill Magazine* 9 (1864): 219–31.

Litvack, Leon. "Outposts of Empire: Scientific Discovery and Colonial Displacement in Gaskell's *Wives and Daughters.*" *Review of English Studies: The Leading Journal of English Literature and the English Language* 55, no. 222 (2004): 727–58.

Logan, Deborah Anna. *The Hour and the Woman: Harriet Martineau's "Somewhat Remarkable Life."* Dekalb: Northern Illinois University Press, 2002.

Logan, Peter Melville. *Nerves and Narratives: A Cultural History of Hysteria in Nineteenth-Century British Prose.* Berkeley: University of California Press, 1997.

Lytton, Edward Bulwer. *The Student: A Series of Papers.* London: Saunders and Otley, 1840. Originally published in 1835.

Maglen, Krista. "'The First Line of Defense': British Quarantine and the Port Sanitary Authorities in the Nineteenth Century." *Social History of Medicine* 15, no. 2 (2002): 413–28.

———. "'In This Miserable Spot Called Quarantine': The Healthy and the Unhealthy in Nineteenth-Century Australian and Pacific Quarantine Stations." *Science in Context* 19, no. 3 (September 2006): 317–36.

Martineau, Harriet. *Autobiography.* Edited by Maria Weston Chapman. Boston: James R. Osgood and Company, 1877.

———. *Deerbrook.* Edited by Valerie Sanders. London: Penguin, 2004.

———. *Harriet Martineau: Selected Letters.* Edited by Valerie Sanders. Oxford, UK: Clarendon Press, 1990.

———. *Life in the Sick-Room.* Edited by Maria H. Frawley. Toronto, ON: Broadview Press, 2003.

McDonald, J. C. "The History of Quarantine in Britain during the Nineteenth Century." *Bulletin of History of Medicine* 25, no. 1 (January–February 1951): 22–44.

Metz, Nancy Aycock. "Discovering a World of Suffering: Fiction and the Rhetoric of Sanitary Reform, 1840–1860." *Nineteenth-Century Contexts* 15, no. 1 (1991): 65–81.

Miller, D. A. *Jane Austen, or the Secret of Style.* Princeton: Princeton University Press, 2003.

———. "The Late Jane Austen." *Raritan* (Summer 1990): 55–79.

———. *Narrative and Its Discontents: Problems of Closure in the Traditional Novel.* Princeton: Princeton University Press, 1989.

Montgomery, Kathryn. *Doctors' Stories: The Narrative Structure of Medical Knowledge.* Princeton: Princeton University Press, 1991.

Morgan, Susan. *Daughters in Time: Imagining Gender in 19th-Century British Fiction.* Oxford: Oxford University Press, 1989.

Mullen, John. *Sentiment and Sociability: The Language of Feeling in the Eighteenth Century.* Oxford, UK: Clarendon Press, 1988.

Nandrea, Lorri G. "Difference and Repetition in Austen's *Persuasion.*" *Studies in the Novel* 39, no. 1 (2007): 48–64.

Nightingale, Florence. *Cassandra: An Essay.* Old Westbury, NY: Feminist Press, 1979.

"Novels Past and Present." *Saturday Review of Politics, Literature, Science, and Art,* April 14, 1866, 438–40.

O'Connor, Erin. *Raw Material: Producing Pathology in Victorian Culture.* Durham, NC: Duke University Press, 2000.

Oppenheim, Janet. *Shattered Nerves: Doctors, Patients, and Depression in Victorian England.* Oxford: Oxford University Press, 1991.

Pelling, Margaret. *Cholera, Fever, and English Medicine, 1825–1865.* Oxford: Oxford University Press, 1978.

———. "Contagion/Germ Theory/Specificity." In *Companion Encyclopedia of the History of Medicine,* edited by W. F. Bynum and Roy Porter, 1: 309–34. 2 vols. New York: Routledge, 1993.

———. "The Meaning of Contagion: Reproduction, Medicine, and Metaphor." In *Contagion: Historical and Cultural Studies,* edited by Alison Bashford and Claire Hooker, 15–38. London: Routledge, 2001.

Philpotts, Trey. *The Companion to* Little Dorrit. Mountfield, UK: Helm Information, 2003.

Pichanick, Valerie Kossew. *Harriet Martineau: The Woman and Her Work, 1802–1876.* Ann Arbor: University of Michigan Press, 1980.

Porter, Dorothy, and Roy Porter. *Patient's Progress: Doctors and Doctoring in Eighteenth-Century England.* Cambridge, UK: Polity Press, 1989.

Porter, Roy. *Doctor of Society: Thomas Beddoes and the Sick Trade in Late Enlightenment England.* The Wellcome Institute Series in the History of Medicine. London: Routledge, 1992.

———. "Spreading Medical Enlightenment: The Popularization of Medicine in Georgian England, and Its Paradoxes." In *The Popularization of Medicine, 1650–1830,* edited by Roy Porter, 215–31. New York: Routledge, 1992.

Porter, Roy, and Dorothy Porter. *In Sickness and in Health: The British Experience, 1650–1850.* New York: Blackwell, 1988.

———. *Patient's Progress: Doctors and Doctoring in Eighteenth-Century England.* Cambridge, UK: Polity Press, 1989.

———. "The Rise of the English Drug Industry: The Role of Thomas Corbyn." *Medical History* 33 (1989): 280.

Postlethwaite, Diana. "Mothering and Mesmerism in the Life of Harriet Martineau." *Signs: Journal of Women in Culture and Society* 14, no. 3 (1989): 583–609.

Prince, Gerald. "Narrative Analysis and Narratology." *New Literary History* 13, no. 2 (Winter 1982): 179–88.

"Quarantine." *Fraser's Magazine* 47 (1853): 74–83.

Reed, John R. "Confinement and Character in Dickens' Novels." *Dickens Studies Annual* 1 (1970): 41–54.

Rigby, Elizabeth. Reviews of *Vanity Fair,* by William Makepeace Thackeray, and *Jane Eyre,* by Charlotte Brontë. *Quarterly Review* 83 (1848): 153–85.

Rimmon-Kenan, Shlomith. "The Story of 'I': Illness and Narrative Identity." *Narrative* 10, no. 1 (January 2002): 9–27.

Roberts, Caroline. *The Woman and the Hour: Harriet Martineau and Victorian Ideologies.* Toronto: University of Toronto Press, 2002.

Rogers, James Frederick. "A Patron Saint and Her Agent." *American Journal of Public Health* 42, no. 9 (1952): 1099–102.

Rosen, George. "Disease, Debility, and Death." In *The Victorian City,* edited by H. J. Dyos, 625–67. London: Routledge and Kegan Paul, 1973.

———. *A History of Public Health.* New York: MD Publications, 1958.

Rothfield, Lawrence. *Vital Signs: Medical Realism in Nineteenth-Century Fiction.* Princeton: Princeton University Press, 1994.

Ruskin, John. "Fiction, Fair and Foul." In *The Works of John Ruskin,* edited by E. T. Cook and Alexander Wedderburn, 265–397 London: Longmans, Green, 1908. Available from Google Books.

Sanders, Valerie. *Reason over Passion: Harriet Martineau and the Victorian Novel.* Sussex, UK: Harvester Press, 1986.

Schor, Hilary M. *Dickens and the Daughter of the House.* Cambridge: Cambridge University Press, 1999.

———. *Scheherezade in the Marketplace: Elizabeth Gaskell and the Victorian Novel.* New York: Oxford University Press, 1992.

Schwarzbach, F. S. "*Bleak House*: The Social Pathology of Urban Life." *Literature and Medicine* 9 (1990): 93–104.

———. "The Fever of Bleak House." *English Language Notes* 20, no. 3/4 (March 1983): 21–27.

Shand, A[lexander] I. "The Pleasures of Sickness." *Blackwood's Edinburgh Magazine* 145 (April 1889): 546–56.

Showalter, Elaine. *Female Malady: Women, Madness, and English Culture, 1830–1980.* London: Virago Press, 1985.

Shuttleworth, Sally. *Charlotte Brontë and Victorian Psychology.* Cambridge: Cambridge University Press, 1996.

Sinclair, John. *The Code of Health and Longevity.* Vol. 3. Edinburgh: Arch Constable, 1807.

———. *The Code of Health and Longevity.* 4th ed. London: B. McMillan, 1818. Available from Google Books.

———. *The Code of Health and Longevity.* 6th ed. London: Sherwood, Gilbert and Piper, 1844. Available from Google Books.

Singer, Peter. Introduction to *Galen: Selected Works.* Oxford World's Classics Series. Oxford: Oxford University Press, 1997.

Smith, Ginnie. "Prescribing the Rules of Health: Self-Help and Advice in the Late Eighteenth Century." In *Patients and Practitioners: Lay Perceptions of Medicine in Pre-industrial Society,* edited by Roy Porter, 249–82. Cambridge: Cambridge University Press, 1985.

Smith, Thomas Southwood. "Contagion and Sanitary Laws." January 1825. In *Public Health in the Victorian Age: Debates on the Issue from 19th Century Critical Journals,* edited by Ruth G. Hodgkinson. Farnborough, UK: Gregg, 1973.

———. *Epidemics Considered with Relation to Their Common Nature . . . : in Two Lectures Delivered at the Philosophical Institution, Edinburgh, November 1855.* Edinburgh: Edmonston and Douglas, 1856.

Snyder, Katherine. *Bachelors, Manhood, and the Novel, 1850–1925.* Cambridge: Cambridge University Press, 2000.

Sontag, Susan. *Illness as Metaphor.* New York: Vintage Books, 1979.

Sparks, Tabitha. *The Doctor in the Victorian Novel: Family Practice.* Aldershot, UK: Ashgate, 2009.

Stewart, Garrett. "Dickens and the Narratography of Closure." *Critical Inquiry* 34, no. 3 (Spring 2008): 509–42.

Strange, William. *The Restoration of Health; or, The Application of the Laws of Hygiene to the Recovery of Health, Forming a Manual for the Invalid and a Guide in the Sick-Room.* London: Longmans, Green, 1865.

———. *The Seven Sources of Health.* London: Henry Renshaw, 1864. Available from Google Books.

Tanner, Tony. *Jane Austen.* Cambridge: Harvard University Press, 1986

Thomas, Gillian. *Harriet Martineau.* Twayne's English Author Series. Boston: Twayne, 1985.

Thomson, A. T. "Lecture XXVII: Public Health." *Lancet,* April 8, 1837, 65–74.

Thormählen, Marianne, ed. *The Brontës in Context.* Cambridge: Cambridge University Press, 2012.

Tissot, S. A. D. *Advice to the People in General with Regard to Their Health.* 4th ed. Philadelphia: John Sparhawk, 1771.

Tougow, Jason Daniel. *Strange Cases: The Medical Case History and the British Novel.* New York: Routledge, 2006.

Trilling, Lionel. "Little Dorrit." *Kenyon Review* 25 (1953): 577–90.

———. "Mansfield Park." In *Jane Austen: A Collection of Essays,* edited by Ian Watt, 124–40. Englewood Cliffs, NJ: Prentice Hall, 1963.

Trollope, Anthony. *Doctor Thorne.* Chronicles of Barsetshire. London: Chapman and Hall, 1858.

Tuite, Clara. *Romantic Austen: Sexual Politics and the Literary Canon.* Cambridge Studies in Romanticism. Cambridge: Cambridge University Press, 2002.

Verbrugge, Martha. *Able-Bodied Womanhood: Personal Health and Social Change in Nineteenth-Century Boston.* Oxford: Oxford University Press, 1988.

Vrettos, Athena. *Somatic Fictions: Imagining Illness in Victorian Culture.* Stanford: Stanford University Press, 1995.

Wakely, Thomas. "The History and Condition of Our Governing Medical Institutions." *Lancet,* February 11, 1843, 719–22.

Waldron, Mary. *Jane Austen and the Fiction of Her Time.* Cambridge: Cambridge University Press, 1999.

Wallen, Martin. *City of Health, Fields of Disease: Revolutions in the Poetry, Medicine, and Philosophy of Romanticism.* Aldershot, UK: Ashgate, 2004.

Walsh, J. H. *A Manual of Domestic Medicine and Surgery, with a Glossary of the Terms Used Therein.* London: Routledge, 1858.

Warhol, Robyn. "Double Gender, Double Genre in *Jane Eyre* and *Villette.*" *SEL* 36, no. 4 (1996): 857–75.

———. "Neonarrative; or, How to Render the Unnarratable in Realist Fiction and Contemporary Film." In *A Companion to Narrative Theory,* edited by James Phelan and Peter J. Rabinowitz, 220–31. Oxford, UK: Blackwell Publishing, 2005.

Wear, Andrew. *Medicine in Society: Historical Essays.* Cambridge: Cambridge University Press, 1992.

Weiner, Dora B. *The Citizen-Patient in Revolutionary and Imperial Paris.* Baltimore, MD: Johns Hopkins University Press, 1993.

Weiner, Gaby. Introduction to *Deerbrook,* by Harriet Martineau. Garden City, NY: Dial Press, 1984.

Wesley, John. *Primitive Physick; or, An Easy and Natural Method of Curing Most Diseases.* 10th ed. Bristol, UK: Printed by William Pine, 1767. Available from Google Books.

Williams, A. Susan. *The Rich Man and the Diseased Poor in Early Victorian London.* London: Macmillan, 1987.

Wiltshire, John. *Jane Austen and the Body: "The Picture of Health."* Cambridge: Cambridge University Press, 1992.

Winter, Alison. "Harriet Martineau and the Reform of the Invalid in Victorian England." *Historical Journal* 38, no. 3 (1995): 597–616.

———. *Mesmerized: Powers of Mind in Victorian Britain.* Chicago: University of Chicago Press, 1998.

Wood, Jane. *Passion and Pathology in Victorian Fiction.* Oxford: Oxford University Press, 2001.

Wright, Julia. "'Growing Pains': Representing the Romantic in Gaskell's *Wives and Daughters.*" In *Nervous Reactions: Victorian Recollections of Romanticism,* edited by Joel Faflak and Julia M. Wright, 163–88. Albany: State University of New York Press, 2004.

Yeats, George. "'Dirty Air': *Little Dorrit*'s Atmosphere." *Nineteenth-Century Literature* 66, no. 3 (2011): 328–54.

Yonge, Charlotte. *The Clever Woman of the Family* (1865). Edited by Clare A. Simmons. Peterborough, ON: Broadview Press, 2001.

Zeiger, Susan. *Inventing the Addict: Drugs, Race, and Sexuality in Nineteenth-Century British and American Literature.* Amherst: University of Massachusetts Press, 2008.

Index

A number following the letter *n* after a page number indicates a note on that page.

www.ingramcontent.com/pod-product-compliance
Ingram Content Group UK Ltd.
Pitfield, Milton Keynes, MK11 3LW, UK
UKHW030031180425
457518UK00005B/20

9 780821 422243